Welcome to the book!

In this book you will unlock the keys to getting rid of your stress. Every effort has been made to edit and spell check everything. On that note one of the keys to letting go of stress in the authors opinion is that 80 percent is good enough because nothing is ever 100 percent complete!

So for that reason there may be a few editing mistakes and a few things might be a little bit ugly in places. That is ok because the information is 100 percent perfect! It will help you de stress. Don't let a spelling of formatting mistake get to you. Move on get rid of the stress and most importantly become stress free!

INTRODUCTION

Stress is everywhere
- At home
- In our relationships
- Our kids are stressed earlier
- It is causing diseases like heart disease and cancer
- It is just too much to take!

The world has changed in the last 20 years; computers, tablets and being connected is great in many ways but it has increased our stresses too! We no longer go home for relaxing time off instead we go home and turn on a screen and do not pay attention to what or who we should pay attention too.

This cripples our relationships with friends and family. We also have more work when we get home, and the stress from work follows us everywhere, in many cases even on vacation!

Many people are faced with insurmountable debt and its not just adults!

The kids are just as stressed as us because they have so much stuff going on! Sports, School, Clubs, and homework.

Stress is a real problem with real risks!

There has to be a better way to deal with all the pressures of life, doesn't there?

How is it that as we advance socially, technologically and emotionally in society that we have created more stress for ourselves and our kids?

Just as the world has changed so must the way we look at stress be changed! There has to be a new model that takes into account the different aspects of our lives Relationships, Work, And Self Care.

By now you are probably wondering if I can actually help you get rid of your stress and I can. I know a little something about stress; I have been a stress management consultant to companies and people all over North America. But my accolades do not really matter, it is my life experience that does. I used to manage 8 people. It was a lot of stress and it taught me the keys to dealing with not only my own stress but understanding and developing tools to help others deal with their stress too.

It is possible for you to get a handle on much of your stress and to continue to grow as a person. By the end of this book you will know how to feel good about yourself and to conquer life instead of being a slave to your stress. If you are ready, I am ready to help you.

In the book we are going to cover a lot of ground:

First we are going to dig deep into what causes most peoples stress!

Then we are going to work through the Super Stress Management Tools that are in the book!

We will cover:

- Work stress and how to get rid of most of it
- Relationship stress and how to be a relationship superstar
- Self-care, because it is up to us to help ourselves.

It all starts with us understanding that we are in control of our stress levels. It is us who choose how we react to situations!

It is time to get rid of your stress so let's dive in deep right now!

Overview:

Stress is everywhere at work, at home and in our relationships. It has caused us to stop taking care of ourselves properly. Because of this we are seeing rising health care costs related to stress and more people dying from stress related disease.

Stress is affecting us so badly that 77% of people are experiencing PHYSICAL symptoms of stress. This shows that we are way too stressed in our daily lives!
On top of that 73% of people feel that they experience the psychological symptoms related to stress! Stress is driving people banana's!

Stress has many visible and adverse effects on us like:

- Insomnia
- Fatigue
- Headache
- Upset stomach
- Irritability
- Appetite changes
- Muscle tension
- Teeth grinding
- Change in sex drive
- Dizziness
- Nervousness
- Lack of energy
- Feeling like you want to cry!

It is estimated that the annual cost to employers in America in stress related health care costs is around 300 BILLION DOLLARS! That is one heck of a pill for companies to swallow!

Considering that 30% of the workforce feels like they are often or always under stress at work, it is not really that much of a surprise.

35% of people feel that their jobs interfere with their family or personal time and this is a significant source of stress!

But it isn't just our jobs that cause stress oh no! It is our own selves, the technology and how we interact with each other too!

Our relationships are falling apart and that is causing stress too. Gone are the days of going home and having a relaxing evening. Instead we go home and do even more work and look at screens in front of us instead of the people on the couch beside us.

Stress poses serious health risks too! It is estimated that 60% of ALL HUMAN ILLNESS is rooted in stress! So why are we not put a larger emphasis on controlling it?
Stress is in every faucet of our lives and for most it is only going to get worse.

I believe that the approach here in the form of this book and my other teaching products is the answer to modern day stress.
Follow it and you can have less stress!
It is the people who use this approach and follow through that will have the most success in eliminating stress in their lives. They will be the winners!
The losers will be the ones who don't do anything to help themselves and think that they will continue to be able to manage their stress until the day they either have a heart attack or end up in a mental institution!

You are probably asking yourself who is this guy to talk about how I can handle my stress? Well my story is a simple one.

I grew up with nothing, we did not even have running water. I was poor and my family was considered the lowest form of humanity in our area.

It was stressful and affected my self-esteem and who I was for a long time. It created and maintained a lot of stress in my life. When I graduated I was the first male in my family to do so in two generations.

I wonder if you have ever felt like the world was against you? I sure did!

I had such low self esteem that I did not think I could do anything with my life and ended up pumping hog manure! I wasn't even any good at it in fact the first two weeks I was horrible. I did not know what I was doing and the assistant manager was always there helping me to try to understand how to make things work.

I was stressed out to say the least.

Two weeks into the job I was called into a meeting with the crew manager.
I remember his exact words.

He said – "Jesse I know you can do this, I am not sure why you are having so much trouble I know you are smarter than this. You just have to grab the bull by the horns and do it."

I had never had anyone express confidence in my ability before, not my parents, not my teachers, no one. Do you know how badly that effects most people for life?

That day and those words changed my life. Someone believed in me and I could not let them down. We worked shifts 10 days 12 hours per day and then 5 days off.

My five days off came and for five days straight I studied the manuals, I knew it was go time, I could work and gain and actually earn this man's trust or I could remain the way I was forever. It was the only option. No more would I be afraid of the world.

Over the next year I became very good at what I did. I became the best pump man that crew had ever seen. My numbers proved it and so did my work ethic. My stress levels dropped and my confidence soared! 2 years later I was promoted as the manager of that very crew. He had moved up to being the division manager.

I sucked as a manager. I had no idea what I was doing. I was good at the everyday tasks of the crew but not the big picture.

I now had 8 guys under me who were stressed out because I was. Yes I knew the jobs tasks inside out but not how to manage people.

I went from a 12 hour work day as a crew person to a 24 hour work day 7 days a week as a manager. We ran 24/7 for 8 months of the year!

To say the least this caused a lot of stress.

I was drowning in the amount of work and did not have a life boat.

I had to figure out a better way to live.

I learned stage hypnosis….

Wait what?

Yes I learned stage hypnosis and hypnotherapy to control my stress.

I even quit the job a year later and started my own business performing across the country!

With that came brand new stresses

It was not only the work load but also running the every day operations of the business and to top it all off my first child was on the way!

I don't tell you my story to brag that I am the greatest manager of stress ever.

I tell you my story so you can understand that I am like you.

I have had major stresses in my life and continue to do so.
- At work
- In my business
- At home
- In relationships
- In my friendships
- In my finances
- All of it!

The biggest problem I see is that the world has changed and sadly the stress management techniques of the past are not as effective as they once were.

There was a time not so long ago when we could go home and relax, but with today's tensions in our lives it just is not the case any more

I want you to grab the bull by the horns

You can get rid of a lot of your stress with what is taught in this book, but not all. There will always be new stresses coming at you. The goal of this book is to give you a basis you can work off of to help you get rid of and manage your stresses long term. There is no quick fix. It can be enjoyable and very fulfilling to live life in control of yourself and your stress.

But I cannot do it for you only you can do it for yourself!

Through my journey I can help you. I figured out how to take control of my life, my time and my work and you can too.

Throughout this book I will teach you a framework for dealing with stress and minimizing it in the different aspects of your life.

If you are ready, I am. Let's start this journey together!

Section 1: Work Related Stress

Chapter 1: Different Categories of Stress!

Stress can be put into various different categories in our lives

- We have stresses we can control
- We have stresses that we cannot control

Those two categories are it but they can be broken down into further groups

- Work related stress
- Relationship related stress
- Outer influence related stress

And we also have stress we cause our-selves because of bad self- care.

According to The National Institute For Occupational Safety and Health 40% of workers report that their job is very or extremely stressful.

In a survey by the families and work institute 26% say they are "often or very often burned out or stressed by their work.

Yale university's survey says 29% are quite a bit or extremely stressed at work.

With statistics like that it is no wonder the stress of our world is out of control!

Let's talk about the stresses we can control.

Many of our stresses are caused by none other than ourselves. Late projects, portions of our failed relationships, and even our daily lifestyle can cause us stress. But because we are actually in control of these stressors they are the simplest to conquer. To put it simply, change your personal habits and your stress levels change.

We will go into much more detail on this later but what about the stressors you cannot control. There are many like: politics, the weather, the news cycle and all the stuff that stresses you out but in all honesty, most of it does not matter.

What about the stuff that does matter but you cannot do anything about, like how other people act, how they are ruining their lives or your life? These things may be more in your control that you think when it comes to your stress levels.

Both categories of stress

Things you can control and things you cannot control are part of every type of stress.

The key is to distinguish what you can control from what you cannot control and get rid of as much stress as possible.

Here is an example:

Joe is worried his wife is not feeling the same passion as she was when they first got married. He does not realize it but his wife's passion is driven by him and how he acts around her. So he is in control of it to a point. But he has not been nice to her lately so her passion has dropped. He feels she doesn't care and it has caused stress between them.

All it would take to fix this problem would be a bouquet of roses but Joe has his head so far up his own ass he does not realize it. He could have made the situation better but he chose not to by his own actions.

And now an example of stress you cannot control:

Susan has just got laid off along with 200 other employees from her job. She was a great worker the company is just downsizing.

There is nothing Susan can do about this. Or is there?

Has she been saving her money for a rainy day? Has she been investing in herself with continued training or starting a side business to supplement her income over time?

If she has done these things it can minimize the stress of getting laid off and if she has not well she is screwed!

If she had taken those steps

She has minimized the stresses that others can place on her. Even though she has the stressor of not having a job at the moment in her life, she has planned a way to save herself the trauma of that stress and can get back on her feet much quicker than others in the same situation.

Throughout this course we will work on different aspects of stress in your life:

We will start with work related stress because honestly it is the easiest and fastest to deal with. Then we will move on to relationship stress which is a little more complicated. After that we are going to talk about self-care and specific things you can do to destress like meditation, hypnosis, and exercise.

I call this the stress management framework
Only by tackling all three can we hope to reduce stress

But there are some big obstacles in the way!
- What if you cannot deal with your work problems?
- What if you cannot deal with your relationship problems?
- What If you cannot take care of yourself?

Only you can overcome these obstacles for yourself but rest assured that I will be there to help you at every step.

In this book is the keys to overcoming your stress and preparing or minimizing for the things that can stress you out in the future. You can overcome all of these obstacles by just following along and doing the work! It does take time and work to get rid of your stress.

We are going to cover a lot of stuff in the next chapter but before you can actually tackle your stress you need to know where you stand on your stress levels.

The 5 Minute Stress Assessment Test:

Look, I know you don't have a lot of time to fill out some huge test, you are stressed out after all. But to get a handle on your stress it is good to know where you are at right now so you can learn to improve!

For the next 5 minutes you should do this test and give yourself a score. It will allow you to find out your stress levels and the following pages will give you insight on how to tackle the workplace stress that you do have.

Quick Quiz: 5-minute Stress Test

What's Your Stress Index?

Find your stress level right now by completing this test.

DO YOU FREQUENTLY:	YES	NO
Neglect your diet?		
Try to do everything yourself?		
Blow up easily?		

Seek unrealistic goals?		
Fail to see the humour in situations others find funny?		
Act rude?		
Make a 'big deal' of everything?		
Look to other people to make things happen?		
Have difficulty making decisions		
Complain you are disorganized?		
Avoid people whose ideas are different from your own?		
Keep everything inside?		
Neglect exercise?		
Have few supportive relationships?		
Use sleeping pills and tranquilizers without a doctor's approval?		
Get too little rest?		
Get angry when you are kept waiting?		
Ignore stress symptoms?		

Put things off until later?		
Think there is only one right way to do something?		
Fail to build relaxation time into your day?		
Gossip?		
Race through the day?		
Spend a lot of time complaining about the past?		
Fail to get a break from noise and crowds?		

What Your YES Score Means:

0-5: There are few hassles in your life. Make sure though, that you are not trying so hard to avoid problems.

6-10: You've got your life in fairly good control. Work on the choices and habits that could still be causing you some unnecessary stress in your life.

11-15: You're approaching the danger zone. You may well be suffering stress-related symptoms and your relationships could be strained. Think carefully about choices you've made and take relaxation breaks every day.

16-25: Emergency! You must stop now, re-think how you are living, change your attitudes and pay careful attention to diet, exercise and relaxation. This is the road to dying from stress!

So let's fix it right now and tackle your stresses! In the next chapter we really get started.

We are going to cover exactly how you can get rid of your work stress and minimize the stresses other people place on you at work.

Chapter 2: How to Systematize Your Work and Reduce Stress!

Work stress is often the main stress in people lives and therefore it is actually one of the easiest to deal with.

Stress is different than being challenged. Stress is harmful physically or emotionally. A challenge is not. If we complete a challenge we often feel elated and proud of ourselves. That is the opposite of being stressed. A good challenge can often actually relieve stress not cause it.

Challenges can energize us both emotionally and physically. It can motivate us to learn new skills and truly master our jobs. That is what challenge did for me. GRAB THE BULL BY THE HORNS. That is a challenge and it made me great at what I did.

Challenge can change over time and become job demands that simply cannot be met and this can cause a lot of stress. However sometimes it is easy to say we are stressed when we haven't really even done the work in the first place to try to be better at our jobs.

It is a tough pill to swallow but many of us in western culture simply are not efficient at what we do. It is partially our employers fault and also partially our fault too.

Nearly everyone agrees that job stress is caused by the interaction of the worker – relationships, the workspace its self and the conditions of the work.

For some people their coping style and personality are the best ways they can conquer stress at work while for others the actual working conditions are the largest factor in worker stress levels.

The fact is it does not matter where the stress comes from you need to make a plan to deal with it and follow through with it. That is the only way you can deal long term with your stress.

No matter the job you are doing there are ways you can make it easier for you to accomplish your tasks and be as productive as possible.

I know I sound like a Borg from star trek but in truth that is all your employer actually wants from you. To be productive, to keep the dollars rolling in, or to keep the ship afloat.

The problem comes in when we as employees are not efficient at our tasks or the employer has insufficient systems to help us become efficient! An efficient workplace is a stress free one.

Systems are what makes the difference between stressed and not stressed at work.

Almost any task that has to be repeated can be systemized!

Yes any task!

The problem most companies and individuals have is that they have not systemized their work. Sure it is basically systemized but not to the detail that it needs to be.

How do I know this? Because I work as a stress management consultant with companies across North America and the number one way they can be more efficient is to introduce systems.

Systems create a framework that employees can play within it allows them freedom within a confined parameter. Kind of an oxymoron right!

An example of a system from my old career of manure pumping is the system to turn the pump on and off.

Step 1. Close main valve
Step 2. Make sure clutch and hummer are disengaged
Step 3. Start motor
Step 4. Bring up to 1000 RPM
Step 5. Engage hummer, open valve and wait for line to fill
Step 6. Engage clutch
Step 7. Bring motor up to 2400 rpm or gauge up to 180 psi
Step 8. Run the line

I have not done that procedure for 10 years

And I guarantee its right and will be the same 10 years from now. That is provided that the equipment itself does not change in a major way. Some parts of this system are designed for safety others are designed for proficiency.

Why do I remember it? Because it is a system, and it gets done the same way every time. ANY repeatable task can be systemized. Just look at McDonalds, they run systems, most offices have systems, marketing agencies have systems.

A system can be as detailed or as simple as it needs to be. For instance a system for building a car has many more parts than one for changing a light bulb. Systems can even have sub systems and those can have sub systems. The important thing to recognize is that any task can be managed when it is broken down into manageable part.

This is the first key to managing your work stress – creating a system for yourself that is efficient for the job and is actually manageable. One step at a time.

90 percent of your work stress can be eliminated with just this one piece of advice. CREATE SYSTEMS FOR YOUR REPEATABLE JOBS! If you do this you have a plan of attack for everything you do and become much more efficient at it. It is not enough to know it in your head you must have it written down somewhere and placed into a Standard Operating Procedure. If you do this and you ever move up in the world to be a manager you will have every bit of your basic knowledge ready to hand off to the new person in your position. This allows them to do your old job almost as efficiently as you do right off the starting line.

The rest falls into the work relationships category. For now let's look at a great example of systems working in real life.

Public schools

I know they are not the best thing on earth but the fact is that they have a system that works.

It is not perfect but in America this system has produced an 80 percent average graduation rate.

This shows that the school system works for most but not all and that not everyone can achieve success with it. Instead for these individuals they would need a different system that work for them

Everything that is repeatable can be systemized It is true.
In my business I have systems to keep my stress levels low
- I have a system for booking my stage hypnosis show
- I have a system for marketing my hypnosis show
- I have a system for creating products just like this
- I have a system for creating customized speeches
- It is all templates and systems that are put into play and that work.

Quick stats:

One fourth of employees view work as the number one stressor in their lives
- Northwestern National Life.

Three quarters of people believe the worker has more on the job stress than a generation ago.
-Princeton Survey Research Associates

Problems at work are more strongly associated with health complaints than are any other life stressor – more so than even financial problems or family problems.
-St paul Fire and Marine Insurance CO

Maybe it is time we take a serious look at our workplaces and do a bit of a revamp on how we do things.

Back when I was pumping hog manure for a living we had a goal. Less than 1 penny per gallon. Over 4 years that goal never changed even though our costs did.

To meet that goal we had to pump every day no matter what. Every day we did not pump we lost money. Everyone knew the goal and we had systems in place to make sure it happened.

I know you are sick of hearing of hog manure But it does illustrate that almost anything can be systemized, even pumping poop!

So what can you systemize in your job that is not already that would make you have less stress and get more done?

How to systematize your work:

Step One:
Make a list of the repeat tasks that you are always doing

Step Two:
Create a step by step check list of what needs to be done in what order to be most efficient.

Step Three:
When the task comes up follow the procedure.

So systemizing things can be as simple or as complex as you want to make it. I know it sounds so simple but most people are afraid to take this simple advice and just do it!

If you knew that by doing this that tomorrow it would allow you to sit back and relax for an extra 15 minute at work would you do it?

If you knew this one task would get you a raise and a promotion in the next few months would you do it?

Systemizing things at first is hard but soon you learn how to do it much better and it becomes second nature.

If you are a chef do you have a system for what to have the prep team do in the morning?
If you are a business owner do you have a step by step system for marketing?
A trucker? You already have a system for when you do a circle check don't you? What about to plan your whole day?

One of my systems is actually planning out my day and it is really not a hard thing to do for me as a business owner or for you in your real life or work.

My personal way of planning out my day is a short form I fill out every morning as I have my morning coffee:

Project _____

5 Things I must do today to move this project towards completion.

1._____
2._____

3._____
4._____
5._____

Timeframes
Morning tasks
9-11

Afternoon tasks
1-3

3-4

Priorities for the day no matter what tasks these get done first period.

_____
_____
_____
_____
_____
_____

You can do this too. If you prioritize your work day and make a list of what needs to get done you will be much more likely to actually get the work that is most important done.

Yep I have a 5 hour work day in my business and any one I hire does too. In that 5 hours I get more real work done than most do in 12. Yesterday I wrote 40 pages of this book in 4 hours. I also sent out new directions to my personal assistant and did some marketing.

Systems have helped me be much more efficient in my business. At 40 pages per day I can write a 150 page book in 4 days edit it on the fifth and with Amazons create space I can have a book done start to finish in about a three week time span. Most people take years to write a book and in truth with systems it can be done in under a month if you know what you are doing.

Even if you are not a business owner or writer there are other benefits to having systems. If you are an employee and you want to move up it is good to have the systems in place for when you want to train someone. The job is literally laid out in front of them.

For employers if you have well laid out systems you can put almost anyone into the position and train them the specific way you do it.

Some of the largest businesses on earth rely on systems:
- MacDonald's and other major fast food retailers
- Walmart has systems for doing things
- Vehicle Manufacturers like boing and Ford have systems

Heck The world famous car manufacturer HENRY FORD created the assembly line. All the assembly line is – a system!

If you have a system it can tell you your input and your output! This becomes crucial for being able to manage your stress!

Once you have good systems you have the basis for far less stress.

How to create a system if you don't currently have a system in place

The Backwards System Building Method- The system?

To create a system I like to work with the end in mind. This ensures you get all of the steps because you have to think and work backwards through them.

- Step 1: Write down what is the end goal
- Step 2: Write down what is the step you took just before you accomplished the goal
- Step 3: Write down the step before the last step
- Step 4: Write down the step before the last step
- Step 5: Keep going until you reach the very first step
- Step 6: Review your work and create a checklist of tasks to be done for this system

Here is an example from my business

- Goal: Book 20 holiday party hypnosis shows in November and December at $5000 each

Working backwards:
- The final step was getting the signed contract in my hand
- Sending the contract
- Following up with the potential clients from my list
- Sending marketing materials to the potential clients from my list
- Sending a postcard to company holiday party planners
- Get list of 4000 company holiday party planners

- Create a postcard targeting company holiday party planners

Then I just flip it over and know my path to success. By working backwards it lets me think through the steps. You don't have to work backwards at all you can work forwards and just ask yourself what are the steps to accomplishing this task.

I know it becomes kind of a paint by the numbers scenario but it does free up your mind from stress when you know the exact steps to getting the job done.

Each job you do inside your work life can have a different system in place.

Systems are not the only thing you can do to make your work life easier. It does go a long way to reduce stress by creating and using systems, but let's face it you are going to have other stresses from the people you interact with and from your own issues with getting your job done.

Chapter 3: Stress and Procrastination!

Do you remember being in high school?

We all did it, we all just got our projects finished last minute on the bus. Well, at least I did and it was never good and my grades suffered.

Unfortunately many of us have taken this same attitude into work, we have lots of time to complete the projects but we procrastinate and just do not get them done on time. OR worse the boss does not tell us there is a time limit at all and just expects them done on his time schedule.

It's kind of like star trek "I need 2 days to fix the warp coil captain" "You have 1 hour Jordy"

Talk about a great way to create a lot of stress at work! Well let's get rid of that procrastination right now!

You have a deadline looming and let's face it!

Instead of doing your work, you are doing things like checking email, social media, watching videos, surfing blogs and forums.

You know you should be working, but you just don't feel like doing anything.

We are all familiar with procrastination.

When we procrastinate, we waste our free time and put off important tasks we should be doing them until it's too late. Then when it is actually too late, we panic and wish we got started earlier.

The chronic procrastinators I know have spent years of their life looped in this cycle. Delaying, putting off things, slacking, hiding from work, facing work only when it's unavoidable, then repeating this loop all over again. It's a bad habit that eats away at us causing stress and prevents us from achieving greater results in life.

Don't let procrastination take over your life. Here, I will share my personal procrastination busting secret steps which I use to overcome procrastination with great success. These steps will definitely help you reduce your stress!

Step 1: Break your work into little steps.

Part of the reason why we procrastinate is because, subconsciously, we find the work too overwhelming for us. Break it down into little parts, then focus on one part at the time.

If you still procrastinate on the task after breaking it down, then break it down even further. This is kind of like building small systems in your daily life!

Soon, your task will be so simple that you will be thinking "Well, this is so simple that I might as well just do it now!"

For example, I'm currently writing a new book (on How to get rid of your stress hmm does that sound familiar?). Book writing at its full scale is an enormous project and can be overwhelming. However, when I break it down into phases such as – Intro – Work stress – Life stress – Self Care suddenly it seems very manageable.

What I do then is to focus on the immediate portion and get it done to my best ability, without thinking about the other phases. When it's done, I move on to the next. It becomes a lot simpler!

Step 2: Change your environment.

Different environments have different impact on our productivity. Look at your work desk and your room. Do they make you want to work or do they make you want to go on you tube and look at cats?

If it's the latter, you should look into changing your workspace. One thing to take into account is that an environment that makes us feel inspired before may lose its effect after a period of time. If that's the case, then it's time to change things around.

Step 3: Create a detailed timeline with specific deadlines.

Having just 1 deadline for your work is like an invitation to procrastinate. That's because we get the impression that we have time and keep pushing everything back, until it's too late.

Break down your project, then create an overall timeline with specific deadlines for each small task. This way, you know you have to finish each task by a certain date.

Your timelines must be robust, too – i.e. if you don't finish this by today, it's going to jeopardize everything else you have planned after that.
This way it creates the urgency to act.

My goals are split down into monthly, weekly, right down to the daily task lists, and the list is a call to action that I must accomplish this by the specified date, else my goals will be put off.

With this book for instance: I have a 10 day timeline to write the whole thing! Yep 10 days for a book! This may seem impossible but it can be done. The whole first portion of this book to this point here was written yesterday!

Step 4: Eliminate your procrastination pit-stops.

If you are procrastinating a little too much, maybe that's because you make it easy to procrastinate. SO STOP DOING STUPID STUFF!

Identify your time wasters that take up a lot of your time and shift them to a different place. Disable the automatic notification option in your email client. Get rid of the distractions around you. Turn off you phones, focus only on the task at hand. Multitasking does not work. It has actually been scientifically proven to waste more time than it creates.

Some people have even went so far as to take television, Facebook, and other media outlets out of their lives completely. It may sound drastic but sometimes that is exactly what is needed!

Step 5: Hang out with people who inspire you to take action. (ME)

I'm pretty sure if you spend just 10 minutes talking or listening to highly motivated people, you'll be more inspired to act than if you spent the 10 minutes doing nothing.

The people we are with influence our behaviors. Of course spending time with highly motivated people every day is probably not a feasible method, but the principle applies. Identify the people/friends/colleagues who trigger you – most likely the go-getters and hard workers – and hang out with them more often.

Soon you will be infected with their drive too. As a Speaker I get to hang out with some of the most inspirational people on the planet and let me tell you it fires you up.

If you do not have someone like that in your life schedule 10 minutes per day to look someone up as soon as you wake up and watch a video on you tube.
Then attack your freaking day!

Step 5: Get an Accountability Partner!

Ideally, your partner should be someone who has his/her own set of goals. Both of you will hold each other accountable to your goals and plans.

While it's not necessary for both of you to have the same goals, it'll be even better if that's the case, so you can learn from each other.

It is like having someone tell you to grab the bull by the horns every single day! Needless to say, it spurs us to keep taking action.

I do an accountability meeting every night with my wife and she has spurred my on to greater things. I am also part of several masterminds and accountability groups for the different areas of growth I want to attack in my own personal development.

Step 6: Tell others about your goals

This serves the same function as # on a larger scale.
Tell all your friends, colleagues, acquaintances and family about your projects.

Now whenever you see them, they are bound to ask you about your status on those projects.

For example, sometimes I announce my projects on Facebook and sure enough I will get people asking me all the time how one of my projects is going.

Step 7: Seek out someone who has already done what you ant to do!

What is it you want to accomplish?

Who are the people who have accomplished this already?

Go seek them out and connect with them.

Seeing living proof that your goals are very well achievable if you take action is one of the best triggers for action.

I always say it is not where you start, it is where you finish!

Step 8: Re-clarify your goals.

If you have been procrastinating for an extended period of time, it might represent a misalignment between what you want and what you are currently doing.

This is called being incongruent!

Often times, we outgrow our goals as we discover more about ourselves, but we don't change our goals to reflect that. Get away from your work and take some time to regroup yourself.

- What exactly do you want to achieve?
- What should you do to get there?
- What are the steps to take?
- Does your current work align with that?
- If not what can you do about it?

Are there ways to start working on your own personal development and success that you can do while still achieving those old goals!

Step 9: Stop over-complicating things.

Are you waiting for a perfect time to do this? Guess what it is never going to happen! Ditch that thought because there's never a perfect time. If you keep waiting for one, you are never going to accomplish anything.

Perfectionism is one of the biggest reasons for procrastination. The best advice I ever got was that 80 Percent is good enough, you can perfect it on the back end.

This applies to everything I do because only through feedback can we get perfection in the end and after 80 percent done we have to realize we need to put things out into the world.

Step 10: Get a grip and just do it

At the end, it boils down to taking action.

You can do all the strategizing, planning and hypothesizing, but if you don't take action, nothing's going to happen.

Occasionally, I get clients who keep complaining about their situations but they still refuse to take action at the end of the day.

Reality check: I have never heard anyone procrastinate their way to success before and I doubt it's going to change in the near future.

Whatever it is you are procrastinating on, if you want to get it done, you need to get a grip on yourself and do it.

Smarten up, If you ae unhappy with today then tomorrow will not get better unless you take action!

Chapter 4: Dealing With People at Work

Work relationships can be a tough thing to swallow, there are a wide cast of characters in most jobs that we perform. From the clowns to the assholes to the people we really like, we just have to deal with them.

These days I am lucky enough to work for myself and have staff that do an excellent job.

However it was not always the case. In almost every work environment we have 3 distinct groups or types of people.

We each at one point or another are these exact people.

The work horse
- This guy or gal is nuts! They get everything done! The boss sends them a task and it just gets done.
- Some people believe this guy or gal is a goody two shoes, a golden boy.
- The truth is they know what they want. It may be a raise, it may be to do the best damn job possible.
- The boss loves this guy or gal because they do a great job. They are working hard and doing what they are told.
-

The Average Joe
- This guy gets his stuff done most of the time. It is who most of us are without being inspired.
- An average Joe is a good worker and generally the boss will be happy with them but they are not going anywhere fast!

Lazy Louie
- Lazy Louie does not get anything done and he does not follow the rules at all.
- He procrastinates, he is stressed to the max, and he is not a good co-worker!

- Which one are you?
- Are you the Work horse?
- Are you The Average Joe
- Are you Lazy Louie

Each way of doing things has stress but generally the Work Horse has a lot less stress at work most of the time. It is because he gets things done and is generally seen as irreplaceable!

Those are just the types of people at work but what actually causes the stress? It is the different attitudes and the interactions between them that make stress happen.

Well it is the kinds of person they are!

1. The Angry Person

The Angry Person is um, what is the word for it, angry. They can frequently be found slamming things on their desk or huffing because something just hasn't gone their way.

It is like dealing with a four year old.

The Angry Person actually isn't always angry though, they have moments where they crawl out from under their angry rock, just for a moment, to play with the happy and not so angry folk.

But that time is limited and they will quickly find something to turn them into Angry Person again.
This person needs as much love as anyone else.

Your care and attention won't turn them into happy go lucky person, but we can learn a lot from them too.
This might be just one of the types of people you work with.
Or it could be you.

If it is this is a sure sign you are stressed out and you need to implement systems and stop procrastinating. If your world is not going in the direction you want then change it. Slamming stuff around is not going to make things better long term.

2. The Flaw Picker

The Flaw Picker isn't as angry as the Angry Person, they're just very cynical and tend to see the negative side of everything.

You could say they're pessimistic but the Flaw Picker is more than that.

They're a perfectionist; and remember that being perfect does not actually exist. 80 percent is good enough in most cases!

Nothing will ever be up to their standards but again, we can learn a lot from them and striving for perfection isn't necessarily a bad thing, of course.

It can sometimes lead to unrealistic expectations but the Flaw Picker can help us to see issues and problems that others might not, which is valuable in the work place.

They are the person you can go to when you do reach 80 percent of the project and they can give excellent feedback as to what can be improved!

3. The Clown

There's always the Clown.

This person often bounds in, full of energy, and can be a ray of light in a sometimes gloomy and ill-illuminated office space.

They'll put a smile on your face and you'll want to be around them because of their energy and the way they make you feel.

Clowns have their off days too, though. Give them space and the time they need to think of new jokes to entertain you with.

A Clown can be a huge asset when it comes to relieving the stress of others in the workplace as long as they do not turn into a bully!

4. The Super Enthusiastic about Everything Person

This is usually the newbie. Or the guy that is trying to inspire the workforce! I am this guy most of the time!

They've come bounding in like they are ready to go change the world! This person is a huge asset as they can enthuse the people around them but can also make others angry because they have become cynical and sad.

5. The Socialite

This person knows what is going down in your company culture, they are popular and well liked, they are the ones who are making connections and growing their own personal brand within your workplace.

They're always organizing social events and are great to turn to if you want to learn about the social activities in the area.

It is good to get in with these people as they can actually effect your career drastically with the right connections. Sometimes the old axiom is true it isn't what you know it is who you know.

6. The Keeps Themselves to Themselves Person

This person is quiet and reserved and that is not always a bad thing!

They like to come in, do their job and go home. No fuss, no fuss get the job done and of course no social events, thank you leave us alone.

We love the reserved types, they are our calm and tranquility in a office storm and are a relaxing influence. They are the ones that we know are doing a great job and just want to be left alone.

Often they are like this because they have outside matters that need their attention more than work.

These people are generally what would be considered the work horse type of worker. As a manager it is the kind of worker I want out of everyone. They sound very robotic but it is not true they are just efficient!

7. The Knows It All Person Who doesn't know a thing.

These are the gossips, the killers of productivity at work. They act like they know everything but they do not.

As a manager I hated this type of person, as a staff member I hated this type of person. If you are this type of person change your ways, being an asshole will not get you anywhere and we know you want to move up but can generally see right through you.

8. The know it all that actually knows it all

This Knows It All Person is the wise one. They have been doing the job for years and know it inside out.

At meetings they will be able to demonstrate their knowledge by telling you some fabulous trivia that you didn't really need to know but that made them feel a whole lot better for sharing with you and that's all that matters.

You can learn a lot from the Knows It All Person and I actually quite like to sit next to them so that via osmosis I learn from them.

This is the person you would go to if you have a question.

We can be one of these types of people or many different types over time. I was once a bad worker and if I chose to work for someone else ever again I would probably be again because I know my true calling is not to work for others. At times I have been both types of know it all and the leave me alone guy and at different times I have been the clown.

It does not matter which type of person we are as long as we understand one fundamental rule of working and having less stress. We can only control our own actions not those of the people around us.

We control how much output we have and how much we are valued by our workplaces. There are a few things we can do to minimize the non-work stressors that happen at work.

Dealing with gossip

The conversation stops when you enter the room. Colleagues shoot sidelong glances as you pass. The office is abuzz but nobody is talking to you about it—because you're at the center of the rumors.

In any office there will always be people who speculate about co-workers and their motives, but when it turns into rumor-mongering or outright lies, gossip can wreck careers and reputations. Finding out that people are talking behind your back at work can be devastating. It can also take a hit on team cohesion, morale and productivity.

To get yourself back on track when rumors start to fly, consider these four approaches.

Address the Instigator

If you find out people are talking about you in an intrusive or inappropriate way, you can address it directly, because gossip may in fact be a form of verbal harassment.

Workplaces must be professional and therefore gossip-neutral or gossip-free. A rule of thumb to express might be, if you would not be saying that about me in my presence then it should be avoided.

The employee should address the situation in a non-confrontational way with the person that is at the root of the gossiping. Approaching the instigator in private and politely but firmly expressing your displeasure. Talking to the gossiper about any potential issues and ask them to not talk any further about them. This includes comments on social media, or to other co-workers adds.

A way to avoid this in companies is to have a digital code of conduct. When there are rules in a workplace there can be repercussions! In fact I ask that all of the companies I work with implement this as a policy as in my opinion gossip ruins a workplace!

Give the Gossiper a Way to Save Face

As part of your non-confrontational approach, keep it light, maintain a sense of humor as you confront the gossiper. "I heard the craziest thing" can be a lighthearted way of opening the confrontation. Or you can try asking "How do you think someone could get that impression?" to see what the gossiper might have to say.

Most importantly, take the high road and never fight gossip with gossip. Fighting gossip with gossip creates more gossip and leads to stressful situations.

I have been accused of having no tact in the past and it is really because I am direct and firm in my approach to gossipers. No bull, as a manager and employer gossipers get fired when I find them in my company PERIOD.

It may sound harsh but it is what needs to be done for efficiency and productivity.

Think About It And Turn It Into an Advantage to get Better

While gossip is often hurtful and not productive at all, there are sometimes ways to make it useful. While hearing gossip about yourself in the workplace is not fun, it is actually quite a gift.

The people who are gossiping about you have just alerted you to a perception brewing, and that perception can spread and grow if you don't take action. You can look for patterns in the perceived behavior and important insights about how people see you. As we all know, perception is reality, and how others see you affects their desire to work with you and give you opportunities. So if you want to be an integral part of your work team then you need to make the gossip work for you.

Report It

This is my preferred method for my employees as a boss. I want to know what is going on.

If the gossiper doesn't stop after your confrontation, it can be considered harassment, Document it and report it. For me it is really a simple matter, I have a gossip free workplace and so should you.

Gossip is a distraction at work, and can cross the line into harassment. Don't hesitate to bring in HR or the boss if there's a problem you can't solve on your own. The majority of employers have an employee handbook that prohibits harassment.

We are here to work and we can party later!

When someone has it out for your head!

Yep there will be those people too and they can cause a lot of stress!

It can come out of nowhere. There you are, minding your business at work, trying to do a good job, when a co-worker undermines you.

It could be a metaphorical punch in the head from a new competitor or a conniving, malicious act from an old friend.

It hurts, and it can hurt your career. So how can you deal with it?

We know that politicking and backstabbing exists in the workplace. Many times these situations exist because workplaces are set up to be extremely competitive, with fewer opportunities the further you move toward the top. It is important to remember that the people you hurt on the way up are also the people you will have to deal with on the way down. Don't be a jerk.

Coworkers are frequently pitted against one another for months or years in a sort of psychic and physical endurance test to see who gets promoted. This leads to back stabbing and undermining!

It's no surprise that relationships between people who actually need each other to get things done can turn toxic when it feels like the hunger games.
Ironically, teamwork is one of the key skills required for promotion, but I digress. Without it your company gets nowhere.

The cause is often poor communication or misunderstanding, but not always. The question is, what do you do about it?

Your instinct may be to keep your head down, do good work, grin and bear it and hope the powers that be will see the truth in time.

Or your approach may be to take on your competitor directly, and match shot for shot.

There is a third option that you probably have not even considered. It is a road much less travelled but worth the trip. It leads to many benefits over the other two approaches. Approach the situation as an opportunity to build trust with your competition instead. You'll strengthen your presence and influence in the process.

I realize this can be difficult when the trust has been destroyed. If they have been gunning for you for a long time. but the absence of trust with a co-worker creates an incredibly unhappy, stressful, and untenable environment for a person. You end up always on guard, with your adrenaline pumping to keep up with the competition in your brain, leaving your best intellectual power untapped and unavailable.

That is not a good way to approach work or stress! If you work together you can accomplish so much more. Finding a mutually beneficial solution is both a selfless and a selfish act. You may never be able to have a beer with the co-worker after work, but you can do your part.

Instead of cowering or attacking, try these ideas instead:

Seek to understand.

Make it a mission to learn about your colleague's motivations. The more you know about what makes him tick, the more context you'll have for his behavior. What are their motives long term?

The adage "know your enemy" has been around since Sun Tzu wrote it in The Art of War thousands of years ago. The more understanding we have, the broader our perceptions and our options.

Often our enemies can become our biggest allies!

Confirm your assumptions!

Take the first step and access your assumptions with the other person. This is not meant as an attack, but a level setting. So you can understand them better.

Share your observations in a nonthreatening way. Use "I" statements rather than "You" statements.

For example: "I'm picking up on some tension. I'd like for us to find a way for us to work better together. What can I do to make this work?"

Even if the person denies, you'll learn more than you knew going in and can plan from there.

Change the dynamic.

Relationships are based on what goes in and what is coming out! You can change the dynamic by taking a different stance: be openly supportive of the other person.

Back them up by talking about their excellent performance. Talk up their work to others. Be genuine! Offer sincere compliments. Don't puff smoke up their butt with flattery but genuinely care about how they are doing at work.

If you knew this person could help you rise up the ladder in a year from now wouldn't you want them on your side?

Encourage regular interaction.

More than one workplace feud has been resolved during a lengthy business trip.

Unless you're dealing with a sociopath, chances are commonality exists between you as well — if you can find it.

Look for ways to work together one-on-one to expand the ties you have to each other. This may start by initiating a "how can we help each other" meeting.

Look for hobbies, abilities, and growth that you have in common with them.

When I was working for others one of my largest work competitors had interests in some of the same things I did. I made the mistakes that most do and actively tried to get him fired. (I did)

It was a huge mistake as he would eventually return and become one of my biggest assets at the job.

Take accountability.

If you find your way to an honest conversation, own up to your part in fracturing the relationship.

You have probably done damage too. Think of what you've contributed and be accountable for your actions. Don't defend your actions as a reaction to theirs. Your actions are your own and you control them so if you were an ass then own up to it.

Keep talking.

It is not just in work or business either but in all relationships.

There has to be communication. Many a divorce, business partnership, or professional relationship has suffered from the silent treatment or lack of communication.

When you talk it shows you care about the other person and how you act and the dynamic you create has a large part to do with it too.

Chapter 5: Work Emergencies. What to do When They Happen and Before They Happen to Minimize Stress!

What about the stuff that stresses you out that you cannot control?

- Fear of job redundancy
- Layoffs due to an uncertain economy
- Increased demands for overtime due to staff cutbacks
- No raises

Well even though these are outside our influence we can still do a lot to prevent them and to minimize the impact if they do happen.

The thing you need to understand is that there is no such thing as security any more. No you are not guaranteed to have the job you do now forever. You could be like many people one pay check away from financial ruin.

There are things you can do right now to prevent this type of stress having a huge impact on you if it does happen.

The first step to understand where you are at in your life. The next step is to make a plan and implement it so when you do have a major problem in life you are somewhat prepared for it. Now of course you cannot take this to the extreme like a doomsday prepper but small things add up over time to keep your stresses down.

You need to have knowledge that chances are it is not going to happen overnight that you don't have to worry about these things as well.

One way we can overcome some of the stress is to save money for a rainy day. I know it sounds so simple on paper doesn't it.

10 percent of my pay check needs to be saved every month…

Yeah right… That money is getting spent. I know trust me.

This has been a classic of financial planners for years and for many of people who live check to check it simply is impossible. I have been there, my parents were there and chances are most of the readers of this book are there too. If you are able to save 10 percent of your income that is awesome and I suggest you start doing it now.

For those that cannot I have other ways to get rid of some of the financial stress and actually start saving a small amount! If you follow what I lay out at the end of a year you could have a months salary. It takes time to build on itself but it does work. Of course I make no financial claims to your success doing any of these things and only have my own experiences to guide me.

A way to be able to overcome the stresses of possible job loss is to start your own ultra-small business. It is part of my long term strategy for financial independence. With just 2-3 hours a week writing eBooks you could make a lot of extra money per year.

You can sell them through places like lybrary.com LULU, Amazons create space or any other online book retailers.

I am not saying you are going to make a fortune doing this but if you use it as a rainy day fund then it can build up over time.

It is called a passive income. The magazines I write today in my niche and even this book are going to sell for years and years. It creates a long term investment for me. This is called passive income and will have huge residual effects over time. Imagine taking 3 hours every week for a year and having 50 small income generators for you every month. Do it for 10 years and that is a real secondary income on top of the normal old job.

I actually do this, I write about one of my many passions, Mind reading and mentalism. My weekly magazine (Legacy Magazine) makes me about an extra 40-80 dollars per week which may not sound like much but it adds up over time. People also continue to buy old issues over time on top of this. The math works out like this for a year:

40×52 magazines/week per year = $2080.00 extra that can be put away or invested in other things. Do it long term and invest it and over the next 10 years it actually compounds quite nicely on itself. It may seem hard to start but the key is to keep going. There have been many businesses that failed which would have succeeded with only a little bit more effort.

The key with this approach is to put it away in the bank for a rainy day. No I am never going to be rich but it does allow me to deal with any emergencies if they come up.

If you are looking at starting your own magazine or writing a book let me know I may be able to help you out with it personally, On top of my many talents is publishing books and products in fact I own Purple Tie Publishing. We are small and much of the work must be done yourself but what we do does work for people in it for the long haul! It is all about consistency and starting small. If you don't think you can teach something you are wrong. It is not hard at all you just have to do it.

Maybe you do not want to be a writer?

So you find something else you can make an extra 40 dollars a week at and you save that money!
Maybe it is going old school with mowing lawns or shoveling snow. 3 lawns is 40 – 60 on average. Can you spare 2 hours per week to do that?

Maybe it is another type of service you can offer? The reason for you doing this is simple, you are then taking control of a major stressor in your life – Money.

It really does not matter what it is just simply do it and relieve that financial stress. In the early days of my hypnosis business I had to take on several odd jobs to make things work and while you may not plan on starting your own business it can be a great way to interact and benefit others.

There are countless ways to relieve financial stress you just have to find them! You could do almost anything as long as it does not go against the rules of your current job! I would highly suggest you start writing or doing work that excites you and you actually enjoy to increase your income from a secondary source..

I am not suggesting you become a workaholic either there has to be balance in your life.

The old saying money does not buy happiness is true but being broke can cause a lot of stress and hardship.

Trust me growing up I would of much rather had money than not having running water.

Create your back up plan now and you will be a lot better off in the future than many people who have had stuff go wrong in their lives.

This is the end of this section and I have a few final thoughts on workplace stress.

It comes down to three simple things,

- Get done what needs to get done on time,
- Play nice with others
- have a backup plan for the emergencies

Now of course in this short book we cannot cover every situation that causes stress but we have laid out straight forward ways you can reduce stress no matter the cause be it personally created stress, outside influencer stress or Stress caused by uncertainty. It can be managed and overcome in most cases!

Section 2 Love Friendship and Relationships

Chapter 6: Building lasting bonds

In this section we are going to cover all types of relationships and how you can be a relationship super star. Relationships are one of the major keys to being able to cope with stress. Having healthy relationships requires both give and take. Understanding how to give and take in any relationship is crucial.

Nurturing relationships to improve friendship can have a major effect on our mental health and stress levels.

Any Relationship works on a Scale that must be somewhat even for all parties to be happy
Imagine the scales of friendship

Each scale has 10 weights on it. These weights get passed back and forth with the scales evening out for both parties

If one scale gets to heavy the other starts to move and it create friction in the friendship. Understanding how to balance the scales of friendship is crucial.

If the scales become too unbalanced in one direction or the other then the scales will fall apart.

But if they remain balanced eventually more weight gets added instead of taken away and the friendship blossom into something more.

Love for that friend, Yes I have some friends I love. I also love my wife and my kids but the friend love is a different kind of love.

Now the question I have for you is are you nurturing your relationships.
It is important that you understand that you are the only person in a relationship of any kind that can nurture it. You are the only one that can guide the relationship. The other person controls their actions and you control your own.

Relationships in life are the same as business relationships.

If it wasn't for friends, I would have never survived some of the most difficult moments in my life.

I did not have a lot of friends growing up. In fact until about grade 8 I had zero!

When I was going through one of the most challenging and painful events in my life after my first girlfriend left me, it was friends that came to the rescue and saved not only my sanity but my life!

Friends were there to give me advice and a perspective on my life and quite honestly to just be there.
Friends were there for me.

They were also there for laughter and encouragement. I now realize that friendship is tested during life's tough moments and it is key to getting through life.

We can always deepen and strengthen our relationships with others.

In this section there are ten ways to encourage stronger relationship with your friends. I suggest you use at least one of these every single day to build your relationships!

1. Be more conscious of your friendships

Sometimes we are so busy with life and family that we forget that we have friends. We need to be aware that the friends in our lives won't be there forever.

Although they may be "just" a neighbor or co-worker today, it doesn't mean they will be tomorrow. One of my best friends actually started out as a direct competitor for my stage hypnosis business!

Be aware that the people you spend time with as friends is the first step in building stronger relationships.

2. Don't take friendships for granted

Don't forget that friendship is a choice, not an obligation. If you don't value your friendships, they'll eventually disappear. I recently reconnected with someone that I had not spoke to for years and it was like putting on an old hat.

It could have ended badly though as he had recently suffered a divorce and being a good friend I should have been there to help.

In today's hectic world, we are constantly on the go. If we ignore our friendships, they go away until one day we wonder what happened to the people who were so important in our lives.

3. See how you can help a friend in trouble.

There's no better time to be a great friend than in times of hardship and trouble. A friend in need is a friend indeed.

You don't have to solve the problem but you can be a shoulder to lean on, someone to share a meal with or help with an errand.

If it were not for this courtesy from my friends during the time of my first break up I probably would have taken my own life.

Often, friends who are experiencing hardship don't reach out for fear of imposing on others. I was fortunate that many of my friends made the effort to actually care.

4. Find ways to make their lives better

You don't have to reach out to friends only during times of hardship. Find ways to add value to their lives. Put some weights on their side of the friendship scale! If they're busy with a project and could use some babysitting time, offer to help.

If they work long hours, drop off or pick up their children, run errands or surprise them with a home-cooked meal. The little things count in the big picture!

Find ways to help your friends and they will be truly grateful but even more appreciative of your thoughtfulness.

5. Spend time with friends

This may seem like common sense but when was the last time you spent some quality time with your friends? Again, this goes backs to taking friendships for granted in our lives.

Understandably, the demands of work or family consume most our time.

Our daily lives may be an endless to-do list but it is always possible to set time aside for friends.

Block off time or day of the week for friend time! It is essential to our mental health to be able to have a vent and reduces a lot of stress when we do.

6. Communicate with them regularly

In addition to not allocating enough time to spend with friends, lack of communication also affects your friendships. In a world where technology makes it so easy to communicate, reaching out to a friend nowadays requires only a quick text message, brief email, phone call or visit.

Be proactive in keeping in touch even it's just to say hello and see how they're doing. The simple things matter!

You must have common interests otherwise you would not be friends so share something you have in common with them!

7. Encourage their dreams.

When friends are lost, confused or seek your advice, listen and help guide them. I told one of my friends that I wanted to be a stage hypnotist 10 years ago and their confidence in me has allowed me to live my dreams!

Many people in life are quick to shoot down someone's dream or passion, but without goals or dreams our lives become a meaningless stressful existence.

Hope can go along way!

Share your passion to inspire others and see what a difference it makes to your life and theirs.

If you're seeking to strengthen a friendship, try to provide valuable and constructive advice to them.

Even if you think your friend's ideas are a little out there, help them navigate the pros and cons of their dream without shooting it down.

8. Make friendship a priority

We spend time on the relationships that matter to us. Never having enough time is not an excuse. We make time for those we love.

When you say you don't have enough time, what it really means is that you don't have enough time for friendship. We are burdened with often too much in our lives but if friendship is important to you, make it a priority.

When you make friendship a priority, you empower yourself to say no to other less important things in your life and elevate the value of friends in your life.

Always remember that jobs, issues and problems come and go. What is effecting you now may not have any bearing on your life in 3 months.

It's always friendships that allow us to be our real selves.

9. Overlook their shortcomings

Friends might upset you or anger you because of their characteristics, mannerisms or behavior.

If they are a good long-term friend and you value the relationship, overlook their shortcomings. Regardless of race, color or creed, people are people. We all have our positive and negative qualities. Heck I have even been known to be a little bit annoying and have no tact!

As difficult as it may be sometimes to overlook an annoying or unpleasant shortcoming, learn to accept it for the sake of your long-term friendship with the person you value. You never know what weird stuff they have had to overcome to be YOUR friend!

10. Limit your expectations

Many times when friends anger or upset us, it is usually because of unrealistic expectations. We expect friends to thank us for kind gestures, to call us on our birthdays or remember our important events. In the real world, however, friends make mistakes and don't always do what you think they should. This is on us not them.

The easiest way to ruin a friendship is to allow this kind of attitude to get out of control.
In truth, limiting expectations of friends will reduce potential disappointment in them.

Good friends are hard to come by so value the friendships you do have and they will last you a lifetime.

What have you done to maintain your friendships? What are you going to do today to enrich them.

Chapter 7: LOVE

The topic of the poets, song writers and philosophers. It is complicated, or is it?

Love just like friendships has a scale and if that scale is unbalanced then the love dies a horrible death.

Imagine love as a new born baby if you will. If you feed it it will grow and flourish and change and mature. Sure it will need to poop and you will have to clean up the poop but you knew that going in. If you do not feed it well it dies.

Your love is like that baby either nurture it or don't but it is all on you.

Love is 100% in your control! Yes I said it. I know many don't want to fact the facts but it is true.

100% of your success in love is up to you.

Yes there is another person but if you treat them properly and they in turn treat you properly then love will flourish. If not well then you will not have anything left.

It is up to you to feed their love baby and them to feed your love baby. If either fails at any point the love baby dies! Eventually the baby does grow up and mature and kind of takes care of itself but the baby can still shit the bed every once in a while and it has to be cleaned up.

Wow yes I just wrote that!

The point I am making here is that when it comes to love we are only in control of our own actions and reactions to what the other person does.

It is up to us to nurture the relationship and hope they choose to do the same back. If they do not then it is up to you to decide if the relationship is worth it or not.

Our own baggage is our own baggage and we should not be putting things on them at all!

All relationships go through phases, there will be good times and challenges. When you recognize that your relationship is in a rough spot, take heart. Great relationships don't happen by luck. There are the specific skills and actions that strengthen our relationships.

Here's your Boot Camp on Ways to Strengthen Relationships.

1. Make Your Relationship a Top Priority.

Relationships are like living things: they are either growing or dying. Relationships grow and flourish when we invest and nurture them. When relationships are struggling, it's often a sign that they have been neglected by one of the parties.

To strengthen a struggling relationship, you must make it a top priority of your time and energy.

2. Accept that Disappointment Will Happen in every relationship.

Disappointment happens when our expectations don't match reality. Two people will always have differences in their expectations. This means that disappointments will happen in every relationship. We have a tendency to focus on the negative and we then use this "evidence" to reinforce the belief that our relationships are filled with disappointment.

Instead why not accept that disappointment happens. Then choose to focus on the parts of the relationship that have fulfilled your expectations and even brought unplanned blessings.

It is up to you to accept.

3. Don't Make Derogatory Comments, Insults & Belittling Remarks.

The words you use are powerful. As a hypnotist I learned this in depth. If I say the wrong word at the wrong time it can actually destroy my whole performance.

When you put down your partner or your relationship, you are causing damage. It may seem like teasing but it may effect them a lot more than you think.

Choose to break habits that damage the relationship, especially when you feel frustrated and disappointed. Use words that show respect, love, and hope. Plant the seeds you want to grow.

4. Don't Stonewall Or Give the Silent Treatment.

Stonewalling or the silent treatment is a passive-aggressive tactic that may seem neutral, but is very damaging to both parties. By not communicating you hurt both sides.

Whenever you ignore, stall, and refuse to participate, you are stonewalling. It is a power-play intended to break down the opposition. In relationships that is plain bullshit.

The Silent treatment keeps the relationship in a "me versus you" dynamic. For a relationship to survive, it must be an "us against the world" commitment.

5. Don't Play the Blame Game.

This is a game no one wins. Even if you are successful in blaming all your problems on your partner, you still are stuck with all those problems and the feelings that come with them.

In my own personal relationship I am bad at this I have blamed my wife for things like the business not going in the right direction or for not doing the things I should with our kids. I have tried to change my ways over the years.

The only way to begin transforming your problems into solutions is to take full responsibility for the parts you play. Stop blaming and start creating the relationship you want.

6. Let Go of the Desire to Fix or Change Your Partner.

The only person you can change is you. Get that simple statement into your head! The sooner you fully accept this as truth, the sooner you will begin to heal and grow together. All of us long to be loved for who we are. When your partner feels that you are not ashamed or disappointed in them. Then they may feel supported to choose to change. Meanwhile, focus on changing and improving yourself trust me there is plenty of work to do there...

7. Focus on the Qualities You Love & Respect in Your Partner.

All relationships are built on respect! Remember the moments and reasons why this person became special and important to you in the first place. Trust that all those things are still true. Close your eyes and hold those moments in your heart. Allow yourself to feel again the love, and respect that you felt. Return to these moments in your mind and find new ones to revitalize your commitment to strengthen your relationship.

8. Believe That Your Partner Has Good Intentions.

Psychological studies have proven that once we become convinced of an idea, our brain will ignore and discredit information that contradicts what we believe. It is called confirmation bias and it is found everywhere from psychic readings to politics to relationships.

When we are feeling hurt and disappointed, we have a tendency to turn our partner into the villain. But if your relationship is going to have a chance to turn around, you must make room for the possibility that your partner can be your greatest ally. Believe that your partner has good intentions, but the information he/she is acting on is incorrect or the impact is hurtful.

Sometimes in our relationships we just need to adjust our perspectives for us to realize we are wrong or to know how to adjust others perspectives to find common ground.

9. Learn How to Forgive.

We have many misunderstandings about what forgiveness means. Forgiveness does not mean you give permission for someone to mistreat you. That is accepted abuse and it is wrong on many levels.

Forgiveness means that you accept that we are all doing the best we can. If we knew better, we would do better. When we disappoint and hurt each other, it's not because we want to it is because we do not know better and if we continue to do wrong on a continual basis that becomes a problem.

Forgive that your partner hasn't learned better ways of loving you YET and begin to help them. Forgiveness means you commit to letting go of the hurt of the past to allow for new possibilities in the future. If your relationship is in trouble and you need to rebuild trust this can be the first step.

This does not mean that you should suffer abuse in any way. If someone has hit you or abused you there should be a zero tolerance policy leave their stupid ass.

My personal story includes abuse and other things that I do not normally talk about however it is good for you to know that in these situations the best and only thing you should do is find support and leave.

10. Learn How to Be Fully Present.

There is a difference between being in the room and being present. Are you constantly on your phone playing games or at the table writing on the computer? There is a difference between hearing and listening. Being fully present means that when your partner speaks, you don't assume you already know what he/she thinks. You ask yourself how you can connect with them and care about what they say. If you are not doing this then you are not feeding the love baby. You are just letting it die!

You begin to listen for what you haven't understood yet. You become curious with their world sincerely wants to learn what is going on. This is a than listening than listening to prove that you are right.

11. Make it Clear That You Want to Hear & Understand Your Partner.

Tell your partner, I know in the past I may have not done a good job of listening to you. I see that this has hurt you and me. I must not fully understand what is going on. I want to. I want to understand who you are and what matters to you. I will keep listening as long as it takes to make this relationship work.

If there is sincere interest on both sides you can probably work things out. If not you may be looking at a divorce!

12. Ask Your Partner to Share.

Ask them if they are willing to share with you? Do you listen to them? Their needs desires dreams goals and stresses?

It is important that they know you care and you demonstrate you actually do!

The little things matter. So share the little things too. Having a conversation that shares from both sides is essential.

13. Learn What Needs to Happen for Your Partner to Feel Loved & Respected.

We all have different parameters for what we need for us to feel. Some people need to be told "I love you" many times every day. Others need to have one-on-one time for at least twenty minutes each day. A hand pat from time to time will suffice for others. Some people even need constant attention. Ask your partner, What makes you feel loved? What have I done that has made you feel close to me? What do I do that let's you know I'm proud of you? Then give your partner what he/she needs as frequently as they need it.

Often I have to remind myself that I need to make a conscious effort to let my wife know I love her. For me I could hide in a hole and as long as she feeds me and talks to me every few days I am good. But for us to have an actual healthy relationship it is up to me too.

For you to have a healthy relationship with your partner someone needs to take the first step and the only one you can control is you so you might as well step up the plate and just reach out. Who knows you may hit a home run.

15. Draw Boundaries That Won't Set You Up for future stress and anguish.

When your partner asks something of you, be honest about your limitations. Going along with things that you don't truly want sets you up to feel disappointed and resentment later. You are responsible when you do that to yourself. Not them. They did not set the arbitrary rule!

Your partner cannot read your mind like a mentalist. Be honest and set boundaries that will serve everyone in the long run. This way you know the rules and you can follow them. I know it sounds mechanical but it works! Sometimes it just takes some ground rules for us to understand each other.

16. Respect Yourself & Express Your Thoughts/Feelings Openly.

Men we know we are generally bad at this but you are human so you have thoughts and feelings and have a right to express them. You have the right to say what you think and feel.

A relationship built on false information intended to please your partner will eventually fall apart. If only one love baby gets fed then the other dies!

Strong relationships are built on trust and respect, which can only happen when both partners are honest with each other. The whole sharing thing again right!

17. Beware of Keeping Secrets to Protect Your Partner.

We are often tempted to protect our partners by keeping secrets from them. It simply is not a good idea to keep secrets in a relationship.

This positive intention often falls apart as time passes and unexpected consequences come to light. It can be very difficult to know when to share secrets. As much as you can, try to be as open as possible.

Between me and my wife I don't hold back. If I did it would cause undo stress to both of us and the old axiom is true – Happy wife happy life.

18. Take Responsibility for Your Own Limiting Beliefs.

We all have limiting beliefs the are the small voices that whisper in the dark, trying to protect us, but keeping us stuck in fear. I'll always be disappointed, Men can't be trusted, Women will only use you for your money, I could never love another.

Your limiting beliefs are not your partner's fault. So do not put that stuff onto them. You had those beliefs long before your partner came along. Learn to identify your limiting beliefs. Be careful that you are not projecting your beliefs onto your partner.

Take your baggage and throw it in the trash that is where that old garbage belongs. Carrying it around can be heavy and not all people are the same.

19. Be True to Your Word.

Congruency and integrity are the binding blocks of love. Say what you mean and do what you say. Trust will be weak in a struggling relationships. When you say you will do something or share what's true for you, your partner is going to trust that is true.

It's ok for you to change your mind, but take the time to catch your partner up to speed. This allows your partner to grow and change with you.

When you say something is going to get done do it and do not procrastinate.

20. Take the Time to Express Thanks and Appreciation.

We often take it for granted that our partners will know we are grateful for them. When we don't take the time to express these simple appreciations, we begin to feel taken for granted. Thank your partner whenever he/she does things that make your life easier and better.

Even if it is a small thing like making a meal or taking out the trash it is essential that they know they are appreciated. Just last night my wife looked after our three month old all night because she knew I have to get this book done. I will be making her breakfast when she gets up and fully intend to let her know what she did is very appreciated.

21. Dream Together Set High Hopes

We enter relationships to build lives together in the hopes of them staying forever. We often get caught up in the grind of life's crap. Take the time to dream together and explore what dreams and goals you both hope for in the future. Make goals and plans to support each other to live out your dreams.

Most of all love each other and express that love. Most stress in any relationship be it work, friendship or love is caused by lack of communication

The simple way to get rid of much of this stress is to communicate openly and honestly. That really is all you can do when it comes to relationships of any kind and if the other person is willing to do the same it is a grounds for trust and building the relationship out.

So grab your relationship baby and feed it otherwise it is going to die.

CHAPTER 8: SAYING NO TO PEOPLE

Are you a people pleaser? People pleasers want everyone to be happy and almost always say yes to everything that comes their way. This can lead to a lot of stress in that pleasers life!

I personally used to be a people pleaser. On of my family members was to say the least a leach. They would ask for money and bash me when I did not give it to them. This affected my self esteem my relationship with my wife and kids and the relationship with my extended family. I would put others before myself and even before my family and relationships. I was what some would call a moron.

I know how much stress people pleasing can lead to and in this chapter we are going to cover a whack of ways that you can stop people pleasing forever!

What many people-pleasers don't realize is that people-pleasing can have serious risks. Not only does it put a lot of stress on you, you can actually make yourself sick from doing too much. If you're overcommitted, you probably get less sleep and get more anxious and upset.

You're also using your resources for a useless task that has no benefit to you. In the worst case scenario, you'll wake up and find yourself depressed, because you're on such overload because you possibly can't do it all. This is where people pleasing becomes a real problem that has to be dealt with. You can use the following strategies to help you overcome your need to please everyone.

Realize you have a choice.

People-pleasers often feel like they have to say yes when someone asks for their help. Remember that you always have a choice to say no. If it is going to effect you adversely then you should probably say no. The demands of others should never come before your own personal health.

Set your priorities.

Knowing your priorities and values helps you get perspective on people-pleasing. You know when you feel comfortable saying no or saying yes. Ask yourself, What are the most important things to me?

This will allow you to understand if pleasing this person will actually serve the greater good.

Stall

Whenever someone asks you for a favor, money, or anything else it's perfectly OK to say that you'll need to think about it. This gives you the opportunity to consider if you can commit to helping them.

Sometimes a good decision comes down to if it actually makes sense to help them. In regards to financial situations is this person ever going to be able to reciprocate? What is their history? Are they a leech and a burden on you? Is it actually worth it to help them or should you let the friendship or family tie actually die? Sometimes that is the right answer!

How stressful is this going to be? Do I have the time to do this? What am I going to give up? How pressured am I going to feel? Am I going to be upset with this person who's asking? Are you going to be badmouthed after you give in or are they going to badmouth you either way. Some people don't actually deserve your attention. Even family members that are trying to get you to do something often need to be cut out of your life completely.

If the person needs an answer right away, your automatic answer can be no. Once you say yes, you're stuck. By saying no automatically you leave yourself an option to say yes later if you've realized that you're available and it makes sense to help the other person.

Many of life's problems extinguish themselves a week later so ask yourself does this person really need my help? Are they worth my resources?

Set a time limit.

If you do agree to help out, limit your time frame. Let the person know that you are only available to help them at specific times.

This create a sense of urgency in them and if they really need your help they will comply with your needs.

Consider if you're being manipulated.

Sometimes, people are clearly taking advantage of you, so it's important to watch out for manipulators and leeches!

A good question to ask yourself is if this person is a chronic leech? If they are cut them loose.

Say no with conviction.

The first no to anyone is always the hardest. This can be especially true with your family members. I know it was for me. But once you get over that first no you will be well on your way!

Also, remember that you're saying no for good reasons. You get time for yourself and for the people you really want to help. Sometimes saying no is more about self-care than anything else. For me personally I have to say no for my own sanity and for my family to work. For me to work on others projects takes my time away from them.

Any time you are trying to please someone it is taking your valuable time away from yourself.

Consider if it's worth it.

When asserting yourself, ask yourself Is it really worth it? It's probably not worth it to tell your boss about his annoying habit, but it is worth it to tell your cousin that he cannot borrow money, or that you cannot help your brother move.

Understand that a no now does not always mean a no later!

Just because you say no right now because of what you have affecting your life no does not mean you cannot change your mind and help them later. Many times a no can be temporary.

In the next chapter we are going to talk about when a no really means no forever and when you should be burning bridges in your life.

Chapter 9: Dealing With The Vampires!

I vaunt to suck your blooood! Vampires, Vampires everywhere! Well not really. Over the course of your life you will meet people that are what I like to call Vampires.

These are the people in your life that are the constant bane of your existence and you feel like you should actually care about them. I have had two major ones – Both were my family members. Those are the hardest to get the fangs out. I still feel guilty about what I had to do to put a stake in those vampires (metaphorically of course.)

So my question to you – Is there someone in your life that drains you emotionally? Do you hate being around this person? Do you hate answering their calls? Do you feel your very essence draining around them? These are your vampires. Someone who sucks your positive energy away from you, leaving you feeling worse than before your interaction.

These vamps increase your stress levels so where once you were feeling happy and joyful, after your interaction with them you feel ashamed, guilty, angry, sad, annoyed or frustrated.

You should not tolerate vampires in your life if you can help it.

Here is how to spot those vampires and how to get rid of them.

The first step is to make a list, I know I know a list but why? Well on the list you are going to put the people you interact with. This gives you a basis to judge if you actually have a vampire.

Next to those names you'll have three columns. First column reads uplifts second column reads, neutral and the third column reads drains me.

Then get busy putting check marks in the appropriate column for each person on your list. If you're having trouble figuring out which column they belong in, think about your last interaction with them and ask yourself if you felt better, the same or worse after that interaction.

It will look a little something like this:

Name	Uplifts	Nuetral	Drains
Bob			
Susie			
George			
Herman			
Tabitha			

Once your list is done take a long hard look at it and see who you're hanging out with. Any vampires? Yes? Let's see about staking them!

I know what you're going to say…
But some of these people are my friends, my family, my BOSS! How am I supposed to just get rid of them?" You have three options on how to deal with a vampire including how to handle it when you cannot just cut them off of your energy supply!
Figure out if you could cut the person out of your life. Sometimes this just needs to be done! You do not have to justify this to anyone! If they are draining you dry cut them off of the blood supply.

It's hard, yeah, but keeping these people in your life is going to drain you and increase your stress levels. It's not worth it. Once you kick them out of your life, new friends will fill the gap.

If it's a boss, find another job with someone you'd prefer working with. Yes I know it is stupid but is it worth it to live your life drained forever? I know, this may take time. So take the time. It's your life, your power, make a change!

If the vamp is a relative like the ones I have, begin curtailing your contact with them. If the relationship is abusive consider cutting them out of your life completely. That is what I had to do. There's no law that says you have to be friends with your family.

Don't get me wrong I still love them for what they once were to me. But the relationship is dead to me because I could either keep them in my life or cut them out there was no in between. Instead I created a group of people who I consider my family, my wife, my friends my kids. I get everything I need from them and give them what they need in return.

But what if you cannot cut them out? Well you've got to learn to put up a neck shield against their attacks so they cannot bite so hard! Never go into an interaction with the vampire until your shields are up and your armor is on.

How do you do this? First, acknowledge what's about to happen. I'm going to my brother's house, he's going to ask for money and I am going to be called every name in the book when I don't give in. Or my boss is going to be an ass to me at today's staff meeting. Then, prepare your response ahead of time.

By knowing what is going to happen you can set up your armor and prepare your response. By doing this you effectively don't let the vampire bite you.

Do not sink to their level. Let their attack hit your shield and bounce off. Do not let them make you bleed. If you do you are sure to be more stressed out!

Vampires only have power if you give them power. If you can't stand up to a vampire, if you can't cut their energy out of your life, you're going to suffer greatly. You'll find your own self esteem falling, you'll stop feeling empowered in areas where you used to feel great, and eventually you'll be a puddle of emotional stressed out jelly and everyone will step on you.

Work on your list until at least 90% of the people on it are in the uplift or neutral column. This means yu will have very few energy vampires in your life and almost all of the people will make you feel very positive and it will greatly reduce your stress levels.

Don't put up with vampires. You're not obligated to be their blood bank.

Section 3 Self Care

Chapter 10: Self Care Explained

Self-care sounds just like what it is. It is how you can take care of yourself to get rid of and handle your stress. It is you that is in control of most of your stress levels. Up to this point we have covered mainly outside stressors and we learned how you are really in control of them. Now we cover your own personal stressors that you cause yourself.

This section is going to force you to take a long hard look at what you are doing to yourself and at the end of it you will find a calendar that you can follow to try each of the techniques in the book.

I will teach you 7 techniques that you can use to greatly reduce your stress and understand that it is you who is truly in control of when and how you can relax.

I have even put one of the resources, - my hypnosis for stress video online free for your use. Look up Jesse Lewis Stress Hypnosis Video on you tube and it will help you experience hypnosis to really reduce your stress. If you are not into using hypnosis that is fine but be aware that it is a valuable tool in relieving stress in our daily lives.

One of the main things to realize when it comes to self care and reducing and eliminating stress is that is does not work if you don't do it so I ask you right now are you committed to reducing your stress levels? Or are you just full of baloney!

Self care really does have to become a habit for it to work. If you only do something one time you are doomed to fail. I ask you to commit for the next month taking just 20 minutes maximum per day to release your stress. I know this can sound like a lot but used effectively you can get rid of much of the stress in your life all by yourself.

In the next few chapters we will go over easy techniques you can use to really release all of your stress.

Chapter 11: Stress And A Hot Bath

Over the years of our human existence it is undeniable that humans have turned to bathing as a form of stress release. From the baths of rome to our modern sauna's bathing has been a staple of relaxation and even community. These days bathing is a more personal experience and is a perfect opportunity for us to relieve our stress and get in touch with who we are and who we want to be.

Many modern doctor's believe that baths actually have healing properties and in some religions and new age practices the act of washing away ones hardship is quite common. I am not going to go into the spiritual realm in this book but it is good to know that a wide swath of culture and society has used bathing as a way to get rid of their stress.

There is actual science behind why baths work to reduce stress but here are the basics, -A hot bath raises bot the heart rate and the temperature of the body. This allows you to perspire and release the toxins in your body. Then your blood vessels also dilate which increases the circulation and removes excess lactic acid from your muscles. In turn that lowers our blood pressure and eases pain.

WOW all that from a good hot bath. Add in some relaxing music and maybe a smelly thing and you have a recipe for a great stress reliever!

So here are a couple of ways I find to make he bath a more effective stress reliever. Ladies you already probably know all of these already but for the men out there we were never taught this stuff!

Please note if you are pregnant or have heart problems you should consult your doctor before trying this. Chances are nothing will be wrong but it is better to be safe than sorry.

How to take a relaxing bath

Step 1. Run some good hot water. Not enough to burn but warm enough to relax your muscles.

Step 2. While running the water add some Epsom salt. It is proven to help with sore muscles, arthritis, inflammation and hemorrhoid pain. (If you have these things you may be stressed out!) It also helps release toxins in your body.

Step 3. Add a scent that relaxes you. Essential oils to the water or incense being burnt can create a very relaxing atmosphere. If you want to you can also add herbs for the scents you want.

Step 4. If you can dim the lights just a little bit. This allows you to create a dream like atmosphere and your brain to know it is time to shut off for a little bit.

Step 5. Turn on some music that relaxes you, classical, mellow tones, are usually best for beginners. Unless you are a metal head then maybe that relaxes you.

Step 6. Get in the bath for at least 20 minutes and relax. It is not about washing it is about self care. You can massage sore muscles while you are in there and this can also reduce stress.

Step 7. Make sure you have a towel or two ready for when you get out. A fluffy luxurious bath towel and robe can go a long way for when you get out to prevent the stress from returning!

Optional add-ons:

- Light some candles and make it more intimate
- Have a partner join you for massage and conversation
- Listen to a good book while in the bath instead of music.
- Get a relaxing beverage, tea, wine, its your bath so it is your choice.

The key to making the bath as relaxing as possible is to actually try to make it as relaxing as possible. If you have an idea that you think you may enjoy in the bath just do it. Now is not the time to feel stupid it is the time to discover what you enjoy in a bath and just go for it.

CHAPTER 12: Stress And Exercise

Seven out of ten adults in the United States say they experience stress or anxiety daily, and most say it interferes at least moderately with their lives, according to the most recent ADAA (Anxiety and Depression Association of America) survey on stress and anxiety disorders.

According to a recent online poll done by the ADAA 14 percent of people make use of regular exercise to cope with stress. I wish it were higher as it is an extremely valuable tool in the battle to conquer stress!

Exercise is one of the many ways we can conquer our stress! Let's be honest a large part of our western population does not get anywhere near enough exercise. ME INCLUDED. We think we have much more important things to do other than take care of ourselves. Meanwhile we continue to grow larger and larger. It happens and it actually causes stress too!

The saddest thing about this is that the thing we avoid -- exercise not only makes us healthier but has the added benefit of reducing our stress.

It does not even have to be a whole lot of exercise in a 20 minute walk we can release the endorphins needed to be happier and reduce stress. It also gives us an outlet for pent up energy and if it is the right type of exercise even anger.

It does not matter what type of exercise you plan to do as long as it makes you feel better and reduces your stress. For beginners I would suggest you consult your physician to see if a specific type of exercise is right for you.

Some basic exercise any one can do is to start walking. Provided you are in good enough health to do this you should start with 20 minutes of walking and as your health improves either up the duration of the exercise or the intensity switching from walking to powerwalking to jogging and eventually running.

It can often be surprising to many who have not exercised in a while just how exhilarating a good walk can be. It can refresh and revitalize.

For the more advanced exercisers you already know the benefits of a good workout so use them to your advantage. Intensify your workouts and use them to reduce your stress.

While exercise is a well-known coping mechanism for stress many of us don't use it even though it is one of the most recommended by health care professionals.

The physical benefits of exercise are not the only benefits but they are worth noting- Improved physical conditioning, weight loss, muscle strengthening, reduction in weight related illness like heart disease and diabetes are all part of exercising. Add to those things the mental benefits of self-esteem, self- worth, self-care, mental conditioning, and accomplishment it becomes a no brainer to exercise to reduce stress.

Some great ways to reduce your stress with exercise are:

Do yoga

It is not only relaxing but it stretches all of those muscles out and you can actually get a good calorie burn going on if it is done the right way. If you want to do some awesome power yoga check out DDP yoga for some tips!

Hit something

Sometimes to relieve stress all we want to do is let out the anger. So grab some gloves and a bag and beat the living shit out of it. Go until the point you are exhausted. This allows you to not only get a good workout in but get rid of those frustrations that can build up.

You may feel like crap the next day but that is because you have engaged all of those muscles and emotions that you have kept built up inside of you.

I am not one to sugar coat anything. Throughout the book you have read about dead love babies, cutting people out of your life and even realizing much of your stress is your own fault. Well the fact is that many of us just want to punch something so go punch a bag!

Run Run Run

For some people running is extremely therapeutic. It allows you to get those muscles engaged get the heart rate up and just let loose. You cannot run away from your problems but running can reduce stress.

Be a kid and go for a bike ride!

Remember being a kid and just going for a long bike ride to god knows where? I do, we lived 12 miles out of town and one time when I was about 10 or so I biked all the way to town. I had a glorious time! It was fun and I learned alto about my self during that time.

So why not embrace your inner kid and go for a bike ride? It can be no only physically demanding but can also get your mental facilities working because you can think things through on a bike!

When stress affects the brain, with its many neural connections, the rest of the body feels the results as well. So it is undeniable if your body feels better, so does your mind.

Exercise and other physical activity actually produce endorphins — chemicals in the brain that act as natural painkillers — and also improve the ability to sleep, which in turn reduces stress.

Scientists have found that regular exercise has been shown to decrease overall levels of tension, elevate and stabilize mood, improve sleep, and improve self-esteem.

Even five minutes of aerobic exercise can stimulate anti-anxiety effects.

So the question is why are you not exercising a lot more? Get up get moving and reduce your stress!

CHAPTER 13: HYPNOSIS TECHNIQUES TO RELIEVE STRESS

This was once my major passion in life. Hypnosis was one of the keys to me becoming me. From my journey starting to relieve my own stress and eventually becoming a stage hypnotist and Stress management consultant hypnosis has been at the core.

Why? Because it works. Simply put hypnosis and self-hypnosis when applied properly can help you to achieve almost anything. I went from low self-esteem pig manure pumper to an entrepreneur that travels the world and have three amazing kids and the best wife on earth. If I can do that partially due to using hypnosis on myself then you can do a lot for yourself too.

Sounds nice right. While I am not saying hypnosis will help you achieve those things it can help you lower your stress levels. I have made a video for you on you tube look up Jesse Lewis Hypnotic Stress reduction that is the title! It will be there when you need it!

The basics of self hypnosis are easy it is basically a guided meditation and the benefits are endless. It lets us both focus on solutions and relax our body and mind at the same time.

How Does Hypnosis Work?

Hypnosis can be used for stress management in two ways.

1st you can use hypnosis to get into a deeply relaxed state, fighting muscle tension and kickstarting your relaxation process. This helps to reduce general stress levels.

2nd Hypnosis can also help you achieve various healthy lifestyle changes that can reduce the amount of stress you have to deal with in your life.

An Example of this is you can hypnotize yourself to exercise more, eat the proper foods, and even alter those relationships that are stressful.

You can use hypnosis to remain calm no matter the situation and when you encounter situations that normally trigger stress you can automatically use hypnosis to react to them.

What's Involved With Hypnosis?

It really depends who you ask. For some people they feel a very distinct shift from normal perception and for others they feel almost nothing. Hypnosis is different for every one and I can tell you that after 10 years on stage doing stage hypnosis and working with people doing hypnotherapy that the reactions people have to hypnosis are different every time. This is a large part of the reason that hypnosis has not been picked up by mainstream medicine (that and pharmaceutical company lobbying)

The basic process of hypnosis for stress relief is simple. You can train yourself to be hypnotized quite easily and in fact if you check my you tube channel there is a video on how to do self hypnosis on yourself at any time even by yourself.

With self hypnosis the process is just entering a relaxed state and giving yourself specific directions for what you plan on doing to relieve stress. If you look up the video on you tube I walk you through the basic steps of self hypnosis to relieve stress and you will even be able to do so quickly and easily!

Hypnosis is an very versatile tool that can be used for everything from relaxation to pain management in the most stressful of situations some women even use it for what is known as painless childbirth. It's easy to do and works.

Hypnosis isn't for everyone.

Some people have trouble getting past their initial prejudices about hypnosis in general, religious views or cultural stereotypes have effected the reputation of hypnosis over the years. Add this to the plethora of people who have done sleazy things with hypnosis in the past and you can see why hypnosis is not more main stream. The fact is hypnosis is a tool and like any tool can be used for good and bad.

How Do Hypnosis and Self-Hypnosis Stack Up To Other Stress Reduction Methods?

Hypnosis does require more focus than techniques like exercise and hypnosis also requires some training, or the help of a trained professional. However, hypnosis may be a more desirable option for those with physical limitations that make exercise unachievable.

There are few side effects with hypnosis and hypnosis can be done anywhere. Also, few other techniques can offer such a wide variety of benefits as hypnosis does.

Here is the very basic way to do simple stress relief hypnosis is laid out step by step: this is the Jesse Lewis 60 Second relaxation technique! What a snazzy name right!

Preparation: Put on some really relaxing music, and maybe light a candle, just like meditation.

Step 1: Lay down or Sit in a comfortable chair.

Step 2: Put your hands at your sides and close your eyes

Step 3: Focus your attention on your feet and imagine a light going over each muscle relaxing for 10 seconds. During each step you should try to relax and let the tension go in the specified body part.

Step 4: Focus on your legs and imagine the light relaxing the muscles for 10 seconds.

Step 5: Imagine each muscle relaxing in your groin and imagine the light relaxing the muscles for 10 seconds.

Step 6: Imagine your chest and arms relaxing and imagine the light relaxing the muscles for 10 seconds.

Step 7: Imagine the light goes over your face and relaxes your head and neck for ten seconds.

Step 8: Imagine the light grows more intense and speeds up going down this time and then back up several times relaxing you more and more each times it goes up and down.

Continue to breathe normally and as you do you will relax more and more and more. That is the beauty of the power of your mind it can allow you to relax more than you ever thought you could.

With training and practice, virtually anyone can use hypnosis, and experience the many benefits this method has to offer.

This is an often-overlooked but wonderfully effective route to stress relief. I truly hope you go look up my videos on you tube and learn how to use hypnosis for your stress management!

CHAPTER 14: STRESS AND MEDITAION – Learning to breathe!

You are probably not breathing right! Well you are probably breathing right to live but not right to relieve stress. How we breathe affects our entire body and there is a specific way you can breathe to reduce your stress and to cope with it better. This chapter may be the most useful one in the whole book for helping you relieve stress with self care.

To see this in action I have created another you tube video you can check out it is on the Jesse Lewis Channel and is called learn to breathe!

The problem with breathing doesn't come from not doing it, we have to do that. It comes from not doing it properly. Most of us are known as top of lung breathers and while this is fine for our everyday functioning it is the good deep breathing techniques that have a great impact on reducing our stress levels.

The best way to breathe to reduce your stress is very deep. To maximize oxygen intake and reduce stress most effectively, it's important to learn to breathe from your abdomen this is called belly breathing.

Step 1:   Get comfortable in any position and put your hands on your chest and stomach

Step 2: Focus on your breath until you feel your stomach rise and fall more than your chest does with each inhalation and exhalation.

Step 3: Breathe in through your nose, hold the breath for a few seconds and then exhale through your mouth.

Step 4: Do at least 10 breaths in a row inhale and exhale.

The time it takes to exhale should be about twice what it is to inhale. The key is to not be extremely stringent if your breath only takes 3 seconds in and 5 seconds out that is fine.

Let go of other thoughts while you breathe.

Do this 3-5 times every day and see if the breathing relaxes you it works for most people. I do mine at specific times I know can be stressful. In the morning with my morning coffee, just before meal time, and just before my kids get home from school. Since I have the newest baby I find myself doing the breathing almost naturally as I hold her when she cries. This should only take a few minutes to do each time!

You can add meditation to the mix as you breathe to make it even more effective. As you breathe imagine that you can see a candle flame, and in that candle flame you can place all of your worries, now imagine your worries going into the flame each to just get burned away. As you do this ask yourself what is the answer to your stress and you will find with time your worries will burn away in the imaginary flame. Stop when you feel calm and relaxed.

There are thousands of other meditations out there feel free to experiment and find one that works for you.

Chapter 14: Stress and Massage

Oh the feeling of a massage is so good, and many of us do not get them nearly enough! I was 32 before I ever got my first professional massage.

Massaging can reduce stress and you do not have to get it professionally done to feel the benefits you can do it yourself or with a partner.

We all know the basics of massage is to rub the muscles and get relief from cramping, tension, and stress. Massage increases blood flow alleviates inflammation and can be a great way to get rid of built up toxins in our muscles.

So how do we start? In this section I will cover 3 types of massages you can do for yourself!

- The Neck Massage
- Foot massage
- Back Massage

First Lets Cover the neck Massage:

Step 1: Reach across your chest with your right hand, placing the palm on top of the left shoulder

Step 2: Keep your fingers on your back and press the knuckle of your thumb against the front of neck muscle just above your collar bone. (We do the front of the muscle first and then the back in Step 5 this gives us a thorough massage)

Step 3: Massage the muscle above the collar bone starting at where it meets the neck and going down to the shoulder.

Step 4: Slowly rotate your head and neck in a circular fashion pressing neck muscles against the thumb as you go.

Step 5: Keep your hand in the same place, then press into your back muscle with your fingertips and rotate your left shoulder blade to loosen the muscle while you massage. Work the muscle from start to finish.

Step 6: Switch arms and repeat on the right side.

This massage is especially useful when you are holding a lot of tension in your neck. Chances are you have grabbed your neck before when you have had tension and tried to massage it. This is the most effective way to do it and is thorough instead of a basic little rub you can get in deep and get some of the tension out.

The Foot massage!

Believe it or not your feet hold a lot of tension and also have nerves going directly to your brain. With the correct foot massage you can alleviate pain, reduce stress, and if you believe in reflexology do some really amazing things.

While this book is not a treatise on reflexology I would highly suggest you find a reflexologist and try at least 5 treatments 1 each week and see if you feel better at the end of the 5 weeks. I know it has helped me tremendously and whether it actually works or not is secondary. I enjoy the 20 minutes of alone time while someone massages my feet.

That being said you can also do your own foot massage:

Here's how to do it:

Step 1: With your shoes off, place a small ball (golf ball sized) in front of you; you can be seated or standing.

Step 2: Roll your right foot forward and backward slowly on the ball.

Step 3: Apply downward pressure on the ball until you feel enough pressure for your own personal preference, but not enough to cause pain. roll your foot side to side on the ball.

Step 4: Place your heel on the ball to make circular motions

Step 5: Take the ball, and roll it up and down the arch of your foot.

Step 6: Repeat with the left foot.

Simple right and this foot massage only requires you to have a golf ball or other fairly hard ball to do. I have also used hard balls from baseball and even my kids super bouncy rubber balls. The big key is to apply enough pressure for tit to actually massage your foot muscles properly.

Back massage:

Almost everyone at some point has to visit their doctor due to back pain and there are a few things we can do to make it go away ourselves. It only has 2 steps.

Step 1: Place a small ball of your choice between your lower back and the wall. I prefer a tennis ball as it has some give to it but a base ball or even a golf ball does work as well. You have to be careful because the smaller the ball the less contact it has with your back and it becomes more "pointed" and can cause pain if done improperly.

Step 2: Find the right spot for the ball, and rock your body – up and down or left and right – to work out knots and tightness in your back. Do it small and you can really target those tight spots.

Massage can work wonders for relieving tension and getting rid of stress try it today!

Chapter 16: Stress and Sleep

A huge part of self care is knowing your limits. Sleep can have a very adverse effect on your stress levels when you don't get enough. Ask any parent with a new baby how their stress levels rise with little to no sleep and they will tell you it is rough. So if you are not getting enough sleep it is time to change your ways.

The problem is that the more stressed out we are the less we sleep which causes even more stress!

When we're stressed, our minds race with thoughts instead of shutting down for the night, slowing down important functions involved in memory, muscle repair and mood.

When we don't get enough sleep, our immune system is not as good as it could be and this create stress on your body! But those aren't the only things put out of whack.

Stress has a way of making us toss and turn — and those restless hours add up to more stress. According to the American Psychological Association's Stress in America survey, 43 percent of adults say that stress causes them to lie awake at night, and more than 50 percent of adults report feeling sluggish or lazy after a night of little sleep. Those are numbers I don't like to see that high!

Not everyone who is stressed is going to have sleep problems but many do. Here are a few tricks you can use to help you fall asleep when you are stressed out!

Method 1:

Do some exercise 2 hours before you want to go to sleep. This allows your body to burn itself out a little bit and in the cool down period many people find themselves sleepy. This will also increase those good old endorphins and make you happier over all.

Method 2:

Breathe deep for 10 minutes. In sleep we breathe deep and it is part of what allows us to enter the sleep cycle. Go back a chapter and do the exercise for breathing deep. It may relax you enough to go to sleep

Method 3:

Play some relaxing music and focus on it while you try to relax. This is a proven technique for helping you fall asleep. If you do not want music try some white noise or rainforest music to help you relax.

Method 4:

Hypnosis! Yes hypnosis can help you sleep in fact I have put together a video on how you can use hypnosis to help you sleep. It even includes a free session. Look Up Jesse Lewis dealing with insomnia on you tube.

Method 5:

Eat a turkey sandwich. While not a long term solution for every day sleep issues turkey actually has a natural sleep agent in it that makes us want to sleep. That is why you want to sleep at thanksgiving after you eat! It may sound silly but maybe all you need to do is eat some gobbler!

There is no scientifically confirmed number of sleep hours we should sleep per night some experts recommend anywhere from seven to nine hours, research suggests that we would be happier and healthier overall if we got an extra 60 to 90 minutes per night. So try the techniques and get some sleep!

Chapter 17: Stress and a Clean Space

You already read my story of how I overcame work stress but I never went deep into how I grew up. Well it was on a farm in rural Saskatchewan (that's in Canada! Eh!) The farm was small and belonged to my grandfather and I really have nothing bad to say about he farm or my grandfather he was a great man from mans greatest generation. A few years before I was born people started dropping dogs and cats off outside he farm and my grandfather would take them in and care for them.

You can probably tell where this is going. Well long story short when I was born the small house I lived in with my mother brother and sister had 50 cats, Yes 50 cats. I am not ashamed of this as it was not me who had them I was just a kid.

Outside at one point we had 60 dogs on the farm. Not good either but at least they were outside.

Anyone with one cat knows how dirty the Satan spawn are they poop and make messes. Add to this a mother that did not clean and children that were never taught how well let's just say I grew up in a pretty unclean environment.

This environment was shunned by most in our area and I grew up with few friends partially because of this. I am not saying it was good or bad or that I even really care anymore but I know what it did to everyone's stress levels as well as my families wellbeing and self-esteem.

This is a book about stress and a large part of stress is our environment. If you have a messy unorganized desk at work it is a sign that you may be stressed. If you have a messy home – and I don't mean normal mess I mean it looks like a bomb went off. Then you are going to have more stress.

On average in the work force we spend 6 hours per week finding files on our computers. That is six hours of productivity we are wasting a lot could be done to allieviate your stress in six hours.

One of the main priorities in the work section of this book was to get systems in place and part of that is becoming organized. Now I don't mean crazy person organized but efficiency organized. Everything has a place and everything should be in its place.

The first step to organization and cleanliness is cleaning and throwing the garbage out. Anything that you will not use again is garbage. Thinking about this I have an old TV that will never get repaired in the basement it has to go out this week.

So what can you throw out? I know you have stuff but what is completely useless to you now. Old clothes are a good start. Do you have a outfit you used to wear back in 86 that made you feel hot. Well its been 30 years and 30 pounds throw that sucker out or donate it.

What about other garbage that we don't see as garbage, stuff that broke that we could fix but don't? Well either fix it now or get rid of it!

Next you need to find places for everything that you do keep. It is not hard generally but it can be time consuming. The good news is once it has a place that is its place.

Next do another garbage run. Do you have 31 blankets for one person? Well maybe it is time to let those blankies go.

Next create a projects list that you plan on completing on an actual schedule! Do one hard thing and then do an easy thing then do a hard thing. This keeps it even and the harder things are the larger projects so it actually appears something is getting done!

Create a calendar of when you will have specific projects completed!

Next you can simplify the space by designating different areas for specific things. Divide the room into areas and work on one area at a time.

In my home my basement has several areas the library, the kids play area, my video shoot area. I work in one area until it is clean and then focus on another area.

You can also label the areas and what goes into them if you have children this helps them remember and is a big help during chore time. An example of this is that I labeled my daughters dresser and closet for where things go. It helps her help me keep her more organized.

Next create a to-do list of things that need to be done to keep the organization going on a regular basis. This stuff used to be taught in home economics in school but nowadays you are on your own!

Schedule the tasks and just keep up with the cleaning, do the laundry and dishes every day, if you have kids get them to help, just get it done. Heck maybe it will tire you out and you will be able to sleep at night in a clean environment that has less stress!

Chapter 18: Stress and Social interaction

Some of us need very little social interaction while others need a lot. It does not matter who you are you need some social interaction. Texting someone is not social interaction it is interaction between you and a screen. Technology while allowing our lives to become much easier has also segregated us from each other in some very bad ways.

Not everyone is the life of the party and has 200 friends (except on Facebook) Me personally I am a loner I don't generally like to socialize I find it trivial to speak to people who do not have at least some of the same interests and I feel more alone in a crowd than anywhere else. That type of socializing is not for me maybe it is great for you.

Stress has a lot to do with the people who we surround ourselves with. There is an old saying that you are the sum of the 5 people you spend the most time with and if that is the case then I am sunk. The five people I spend the most time with are 3 kids my wife and a magician! While I don't think the old 5 people myth is completely true I do think the people we surround ourselves with play a large part in our stress levels.

If you are feeling lonely and uncared for it is not the time to hide it is time to reach out and find others that you can talk to that revitalize and refresh you.

If you don't want to actually talk to someone but just want to feel close to others consider a social activity where you do not even have to talk to people like going to a movie.

If you yearn to make friends with similar interests see if you can join a book club that focuses on the specific books you like or join a team sport on a recreational level and kill two stressors with one stone.

There is also the possibility that maybe all you need to do is reach out to the people you already know.

If you are part of a religious group talk to them and find fellowship.

If you really feel alone in the world and it is stressing you out you can always find support somewhere if nothing else talk to a counselor. I have on my journey and you can too. There is no shame in asking for help in fact it takes courage to acknowledge that sometimes we just need a person to talk to.

When it comes to your stress levels and social interaction just like anything else you are in full control at all times! It can be hard to reach out to others if you need some social time but if you don' do it the consequences are often much worse. The stress leads to sadness and depression. So stop the cycle and go talk to someone!

Chapter 19: Stress And How You Talk To Yourself

A large part of how we feel about ourselves is related to stress and I don't think that this is covered enough in any other stress product. I don't think many of the authors understand how self-esteem can affect stress levels.

For a long time I considered myself human garbage and that I would never succeed. It was not until someone else had faith in me that I realized I could do literally anything. Yesterday means nothing.

Most of our self-worth issues can go away by you knowing this one simple concept. You are good enough! Yep you are fine just the way you are and there is no need to improve unless you choose too and even then generally all you have to do is improve your mindset.

Do you really think a guy that grew up without running water with 50 cats and 50 dogs should have ever become a successful stage entertainer, speaker and author? Probably not. I am not highly educated, I am not anything special. I just choose to believe that I am the best person I can be and always go for improving myself rather being caught as a victim of circumstance.

So this chapter is really about you allowing yourself to know you can do anything. Want to become mayor then do it. Want to be a rock star then do it. Recently I started training to become a professional wrestler. I am never going to be a wwe superstar but I may just make myself happier by following a dream.

It isn't the destination it is often the journey that makes us happiest. The journey of going for something and then accomplishing the small things on the way to the big goal. Sure it is great to achieve the big goal but for some of us like me and you the big goal is actually unattainable.

For your stress levels to improve you should begin looking for opportunities in life and taking a chance. You may get burned but you may also soar!

Talk to yourself in tones of actually accomplishing your goal. There is the old mantra I am getting better every day in every way and if it is not true it should be. So start to get better or end up an old lady with 50 cats and 50 dogs on a farm without plumbing!

Chapter 20: Stress And Diet

Diet may have a larger effect on your stress levels than you think. If we eat garbage we feel like garbage and our bodies are meant to be healthy.

It can be hard in this world of fast food, chain restaurants, and convenience stores to eat properly but it can be done.

Stress levels have been linked to many foods and some of the top offenders are in almost everything we eat.

The top offenders are
- Refined Sugar
- Salt or sodium
- Alcohol
- Caffeine

It is wise to reduce the amount of these a person takes in! Even as a stress management consultant I am just now making my morning cup of coffee! Sure is gives me a quick jolt to get me started but drinking it all day can cause us to stress out.

Caffeine:

Caffeine stimulates our nervous system and too much can lead to a rapid heartbeat, increase in bloodpressure and irritability. Sounds like a pretty good stressor to me.

It also irritates the digestive system and is a natural laxative. It interferes with sleep and can in some cases trigger dehydration! This can kill your energy levels and cause headaches!

Refined Sugar

Not only are sugary foods typically lacking in the nutrients department, but the fluctuations they cause in blood sugar and insulin levels can lead to irritability, poor concentration and moodiness!

If you've ever overindulged in sugary goodies, you've probably experienced the moods swings associated with a brief sugar high, followed by a crash.

One of my many mentors over the years is Sugar Free Barry look him up at 30dayssugarfree.com and you may be surprised if you choose to take the challenge. I did and lost 15 pounds in a month. It made me healthier and happier all at the same time.

Barry talks about how if you remove just the refined sugars out of your life (cane sugar, corn syrups, and 50 other secret names) how you can be healthier too.

It is not about the big bad sugar industry it is about your health. I trust Barry. He is one of the many who have said you can do anything to me over the years and he should know he has been the world juggling champion 4 times! That is a winner to me.

High-Sodium/Salt

Fluid is attracted to sodium like a magnet, so when you take in extra sodium, you'll retain more fluid. This fluid puts more work on your heart, ups your blood pressure, and leads to bloating, water retention and puffiness, all of which are side effects that can drain your energy and increase your stress level. Salt is one bad mother F-er

It can be hard to reduce your intake of salt but it can be done. It is used to enhance the flavor of almost everything. I would suggest the biggest way to combat salt is to read the label and understand what you are eating. If it is a stressor maybe you should limit your intake.

Alcohol

Oh my old friend, the one who makes me do stupid things, depletes my self esteem and makes me feel like crap the next day. Yep that old friend.

One drink every once in a while may actually reduce stress but for many of us we don't know our limits. If you drink to much it can actually add to your stress levels. Alcohol stimulates the hormones that the body normally makes under stress. Studies show alcohol and stress actually feed each other. Alcohol prolongs feelings of tension brought on by stress and can spike cravings for more alcohol. Maybe this guy is not my friend after all.

So what's the good news? Well, some foods can have the exact opposite effect, to reduce stress and help take the edge off. It just goes to show that eating the right foods can help. Some of those foods are:

1: Green leafy vegetables: Just what you did not want to hear. These veggies help your body produce the stress fighting chemicals in your brain!

2. Turkey breast: This produces tryptophan it is an amino acid that helps produce dopamine a stress buster!

3. Fermented foods: Gut flora can have a horrible effect on your stress levels and by eating fermented foods like yogurt you can help to make that flora strong. While this does not have a huge effect on actual stress levels it does help to combat things caused by stress like ulcers and heartburn. One of the keys for this to work is that you use as organic or as non-processed as possible. There is no point to adding a bunch of refined sugar along with your yogurt as it can actually have a negative effect.

4. Fish: Omega 3's can have a major effet on your brains health and are a great way to improve your well being. If you don't like fish take a supplement. Some studies have shown a 20 percent reduction in anxiety with people who take omega 3's.

5. Blueberries: These are full of antioxidants those help your brain produce dopamine and reduce stress

6. Pistachios: These improve your vascular constriction and open up your circulation. Better blood flow means that your body is getting everything it needs where and when it needs it. This can lead to a reduction in stress.

7. Dark chocolate: Dark Chocolate produces a neurotransmitter that blocks feelings of depression and pain! The dark chocolate also has chemicals which aid in prolonging the block. There are some studies that suggest that chocolate could be used as a new form of anti-anxiety drug.

8. Avocado: Avocado's provide 20 essential nutrients. Eating just half of a fresh avocado with your lunch may help you feel more full than normal. It is a great weight loss aid, They are also helpful in regulating blood sugar levels. Put it all together and you have a stress killing super food!

The big key when it comes to diet is to understand you are in full control at all times of what you put into your body. Being healthy is a choice that all of us have. You can choose to put a bag of chips in your body or you could choose to have an avocado it is up to you.

You are in control of you and not anyone else! Please talk to your doctor or other medical professionals before you change your diet!

Some people find it very hard to keep on track with any diet over the years I have done the same I am just like anyone else! The key to having a successful diet in any form in my opinion is to have a plan. I would highly suggest that you create a meal plan at least a week at a time.

Section 4: Your Life And Finding A Balance And Putting It All Together!

Chapter 21: Your Next Week of Stress Busting!

Because this book is all about how you can bust your own stress for the next week I have created a basic schedule of self care that you can follow to actually try out the techniques described in the previous chapter here is your stress busting week!

Day 1: 20 minute stress bath!

Take a hot bath, relax your muscles and reflect on the good things you have in life.

Day 2: It is time to try a 5 minute meditation total time 10 minutes!

Grab your computer and go to my you tube channel!
Do a search for Jesse Lewis Meditation for Stress! It is a
full 5 minute guided meditation that you can use a few
times and then be able to do yourself! Simple and
effective stress relief!

3: 20 minute diet plan!

You need to bust some stress well its time to create a
meal plan for the next 7 days today! Just for one meal though
Supper! People often say that breakfast is the most important
meal but they are wrong supper is! It is the time when you are
supposed to be allowed to relax and feel good and calm
down! So use this time to do just that!

Day 4: Revisit what is good in your life! 20 minutes.

By focusing on the good and not the bad we can be
thankful. During this 20 minutes write down 2 things you
want to accomplish in the next year! They can be big or small
it does not matter. Once you have them written down work
backwards on the tasks you actually need to do to accomplish
them. Do not be vague get specific on the exact things you
need to do to get ahead of the game and from here on out you
just have to do the work to get there.

Day 5: Social interaction! At least 20 minute visit with
an old friend.

Today you reach out into the great beyond and interact with someone. If you have someone you have been meaning to talk to for the last 5 years it is time to call them up! Or maybe it is just connecting with a loved one you need to connect with. The social interaction is up to you but you need to actively do it. Don't sit on your laurels either go out or if you have to invite someone over and share a coffee or tea and actually care about someone externally! Doing this shows not only you care but causes others to care about you too!

Day 6: Create a clean space!

Maybe you should have done this one before the social interaction! Whatever today is the day to find a few things that have been disorganized and clean it up! Maybe you are a junk drawer specialist like me or a closet junk hider like my wife well throw off those labels and clean up your space! You have 30 minutes to do it! That is all after that you have to meditate for 5 minutes on how much a good clean space makes you feel better!

Day 7: Exercise!

Today is your day to get up get out and go for some exercise. For those who are out of shape like me a 20 minute walk is enough to get started! For those in better shape well you already know what you need to do! Consult your doctor before you do anything you would not normally do.

That is it, for the next 7 days you have your stress plan laid out

Conclusion: Stress and the rest of your life

Repeat after me: MY STRESS IS MOSTLY CAUSED BY ME

Yep I said it you cause your own stress! It is true and you can get rid of most of it by making systems that work in your life. Over the years as a business owner and even back when I was managing people I learned that if there is a system in place and I work that system then stuff gets done. If there is no system and no accountability then nothing will get done. It is human nature to put things off and lounge around and do nothing until it needs to get done. We could learn from the bee's they have a few months every year to collect enough honey to live off of for the entire winter. If we were as smart as them we would over the course of the next few months recognize that we are the true masters of our own destinies and can accomplish anything we just have to actually try and do it.

I don't care what your background is just let it go, bad relationships let it go, no money go get some, kids are assholes – don't raise assholes, the batman beat you up in a dark ally don't be a joker. You are in control of your own darn stress so own up to it and recognize it is your own fault. Once you recognize it is your fault you can actually start working on it.

From here on out you have the techniques and the knowhow. If you are truly serious over the coming months you can change your life in regards to stress but if you are not committed then you are going to languish and do nothing. We do not want that do we! Smarten up and do the work you need to do to be happy.

I believe in you! You can do this, get stress free and create your own destiny!

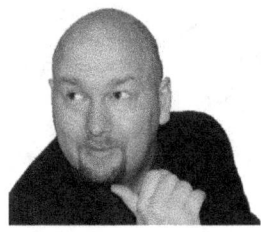

Jesse Lewis is one good looking man! Author, Speaker, Entertainer, and all around fantastic guy!

To book Jesse for one of your events you can contact him directly at jesselewis.net

He speaks on topics like:

Personal motivation
Stress management
Achieving what seems impossible
Systemizing your business and sales processes

And of course he still performs his motivational Comedy Hypnosis Show all over North America! For availability in other countries contact him directly!

Notes: This section is included so you can have one place to put notes and go back again and again. This book is kept short for a reason, you can keep it out on your coffee table and read it and take action. That is a big factor in getting rid of your stress!

_____

_____

_____

_____

_____

_____

_____

_____

_____

_____

_____

_____

_____

_____

_____

_____

_____

_____

_____

_____

_____

_____

_____

_____

_____

_____

_____

That is it – Visit me online at Jesselewis.net!

www.ingramcontent.com/pod-product-compliance
Lightning Source LLC
Chambersburg PA
CBHW070140290526
45789CB00002B/562